730 S. Harrison ST.
Kittanning, PA. 16201
(h) 724-543-1397
(w) 412-648-9449

Pocket Guide to Micronutrients in Health and Disease

Michael Zimmermann, M.D.
Senior Scientist
Director of Postgraduate Studies
The Laboratory for Human Nutrition
Swiss Federal Institute of Technology
Zürich, Switzerland

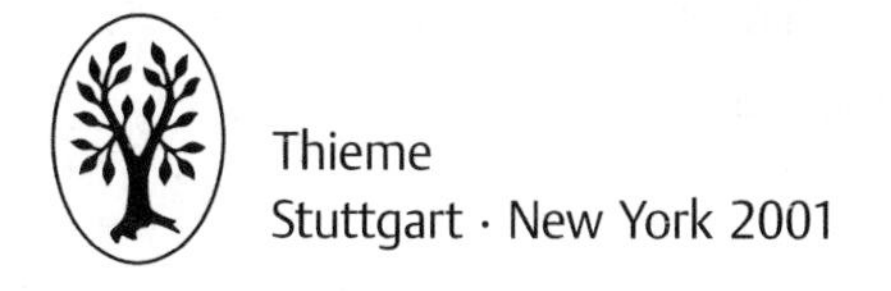

Library of Congress Cataloging-in-Publication Data
is available from the publisher

German edition published 1999 by Karl F. Haug Verlag, Hüthig Medizin-Verlage GmbH & Co. KG, Heidelberg.
Title of the German edition: Bürgersteins Mikronährstoffe in der Medizin: Prävention und Therapie – ein Kompendium.

Important Note: Medicine is an ever-changing science undergoing continual development. Research and clinical experience are continually expanding our knowledge, in particular our knowledge of proper treatment and drug therapy. Insofar as this book mentions any dosage or application, readers may rest assured that the authors, editors, and publishers have made every effort to ensure that such references are in accordance with *the state of knowledge at the time of production of the book.*

Nevertheless, this does not involve, imply, or express any guarantee or responsibility on the part of the publishers in respect to any dosage instructions and forms of application stated in the book. Every user is requested to examine carefully the manufacturer's leaflets accompanying each drug and to check, if necessary in consultation with a physician or specialist, whether the dosage schedules mentioned therein or the contraindications stated by the manufacturer differ from the statements made in the present book. Such examination is particularly important with drugs that are either rarely used or have been newly released on the market. **Every dosage schedule or every form of application used is entirely at the user's own risk and responsibility.** The authors and publishers request every user to report to the publishers any discrepancies or inaccuracies noticed.

Rüdigerstrasse 14, 70469 Stuttgart, Germany
Thieme New York, 333 Seventh Avenue,
New York, N.Y. 10001, USA

Typesetting by primustype Robert Hurler GmbH, 73274 Notzingen, Germany

Printed in Germany by Druckhaus Götz, Ludwigsburg

ISBN 3-13-127941-9 (GTV)
ISBN 1-58890-043-6 (TNY) 1 2 3 4 5 6

Preface

As a medical doctor focusing on metabolism and nutrition, many colleagues have asked me where they could find reliable information on vitamins and minerals and their potential application in prevention and therapy. Literature in this area is often of two types: on the one hand, skeptical and stubbornly conservative; on the other, biased and unsubstantiated. This book aims for the middle. In writing it, I have tried to be objective, but also open-minded. The therapeutic indications are evidence-based, drawing from the scientific literature, as well as my own clinical experience.

This book is intended as a quick reference for doctors and other health professions allied to medicine. It is purposefully brief. Although micronutrients are generally available over the counter, interested members of the public should consult with their doctor or pharmacist. Nutrition and metabolism are complex and individual. Prudent use of micronutrients as therapy should always be medically supervised.

Zürich, October 2000 *Michael Zimmermann*

Note:
The indications for and dosages of micronutrients recommended in this book conform to practices at the present time. Adult doses are given as a gauge of the maximum dose commonly used, and do not apply to children. Every attempt has been made to ensure accuracy, but new investigations and experience will alter present practice. It is recommended that the package insert and/or manufacturer's information for micronutrient supplements always be consulted before use.

Contents

I. The Micronutrients

II. Micronutrient Supplementation Through the Lifecycle

III. Prevention and Therapy

Appendix

I. The Micronutrients

In the following section, these are the sources for the recommended daily intakes:

- UK Reference Nutrient Intakes (RNI):
  Reference Nutrient Intakes and Safe Intakes, United Kingdom (UK). From: Report on Health and Social Subjects: No. 41, Dietary Reference Values for Food Energy and Nutrients for the United Kingdom, Report of the Panel on Dietary Reference Values of the Committee on Medical Aspects of Food Policy. London: Her Majesty's Stationary Office: 1991.
- US Recommended Dietary Allowances/Dietary Reference Intakes (RDA/DRI):
  Institute of Medicine, Food, and Nutrition Board. *Dietary Reference Intakes for Vitamin C, Vitamin E, Selenium and Beta-Carotene, and other Carotenoids*. Washington DC: National Academy Press; 2000.
  Institute of Medicine, Food, and Nutrition Board. *Dietary Reference Intakes for Thiamin, Riboflavin, Niacin, Vitamin B6, Folate, Vitamin B12, Pantothenic Acid, Biotin and Choline*. Washington DC: National Academy Press; 1998.
  Institute of Medicine, Food, and Nutrition Board. *Dietary Reference Intakes for Calcium, Phosphorus, Magnesium, Vitamin D, and Fluoride*. Washington DC: National Academy Press; 1997.
  National Research Council (US). Subcommittee on the 10th Edition of the RDAs. Food and Nutrition Board, Commission on Life Sciences. *Recommended Dietary Allowances*. 10th ed. Washington DC: National Academy Press; 1989.
- Werbach MR. *Nutritional Influences on Illness*. New Canaan: Keats Publishing; 1990.
  Werbach MR. *Textbook of Nutritional Medicine*. Tarzana: Third Line Press; 1999.

The following are the sources for the recommendations on toxicity:

- Lowest Observed Adverse Effect Levels for Vitamins and Minerals (LOAEL): These are the thresholds for daily micronutrient intake at which potential for toxicity exists. Doses below this threshold are generally regarded as safe.
  Hathcock JN. *Vitamins and Mineral Safety*. Washington DC, Council for Responsible Nutrition, 1997.
  Hathcock JN. Vitamins and minerals: efficacy and safety. *Am J Clin Nutr.* 1997; 66:427–437.
- Tolerable Upper Intake Levels (UL): These are the maximum levels of daily intake that are likely to pose no risk of adverse effects.
  Institute of Medicine, Food, and Nutrition Board. *Dietary Reference Intakes for Vitamin C, Vitamin E, Selenium and Beta-Carotene,*

and other Carotenoids. Washington DC: National Academy Press; 2000.

Institute of Medicine, Food, and Nutrition Board. *Dietary Reference Intakes for Thiamin, Riboflavin, Niacin, Vitamin B6, Folate, Vitamin B12, Pantothenic Acid, Biotin and Choline*. Washington DC: National Academy Press; 1998.

Institute of Medicine, Food, and Nutrition Board. *Dietary Reference Intakes for Calcium, Phosphorus, Magnesium, Vitamin D and Fluoride.* Washington DC: National Academy Press; 1997.

The Vitamins

Biotin

Nomenclature

Formerly termed vitamin H

Functions

- Glucose synthesis (gluconeogenesis)
- Synthesis and breakdown of fatty acids (e.g., conversion of linoleic acid to eicosanoids)
- Amino acid metabolism
- Cell division and growth

Increased Risk of Deficiency

- Pregnancy and lactation
- Medications: anticonvulsants, antibiotics
- Chronic dieting for weight loss
- Consumption of raw eggs (which contain avidin, a biotin-binding protein)

Signs and Symptoms of Deficiency

- Anorexia and nausea
- Myalgias
- Numbness and tingling in the extremities
- Flaky, reddened patches on the skin, especially around the nose and mouth
- Hair loss and baldness
- Immune deficiency
- Changes in mental status, depression, fatigue, anxiety
- Increased serum cholesterol and bilirubin
- Seizures; developmental delays (in infants with inherited metabolic defects)

Laboratory Measurement of Status

Measure	Values	Comment
Plasma biotin	Levels <1.02 nmol/L may indicate deficiency.	Literature values are variable and inconsistent.
Urinary biotin	Normal levels are 35±14 nmol/day.	

Good Dietary Sources

Food	Serving Size	μg
Calf liver	100 g	75
Soybeans	100 g	60
Brewer's yeast	30 g	30
Whole wheat	50 g	22
Oatmeal	100 g	20

Small amounts of biotin are synthesized by intestinal bacteria and may contribute to nutritional requirements.

Recommended Daily Intakes

Prevention of Deficiency			Therapeutic Dose Range
	UK RNI (1991)	USA DRI (1998)	Werbach (1990/99)
Men	10–200 μg	30 μg	300–3000 μg
Women*	10–200 μg	30 μg	300–3000 μg

* excluding pregnant or lactating women

Preferred Form, Bioavailability, and Dosing

Biotin	Take between or with meals, preferably with the dose divided throughout the day.

Toxicity

Hathcock LOAEL (1997)	USA UL (1998)
None established	None established

Biotin appears to be nontoxic, even at chronic oral doses >60 mg/day.

Folic Acid

Nomenclature

Folic acid (pteroyl glutamic acid) is the parent compound of a family of naturally-occurring derivatives known as folates. Folate is the generic term for compounds that exhibit the biological activity of folic acid.

Functions

- DNA and RNA synthesis in growing and dividing cells
- Synthesis of structural and functional proteins
- Interconversion of amino acids (e.g., detoxification of homocysteine to methionine)
- Fetal growth and development (particularly formation of the central nervous system)

Increased Risk of Deficiency

- Diets low in green, leafy vegetables and whole grains
- Medications: aspirin, antacids, oral contraceptive pills, antibiotics
- Cigarette smoking
- Chronic diseases (psoriasis, anemia, liver disease, cancer)
- Fever, infections, trauma, surgery, burns
- Rapid growth: pregnancy, lactation, childhood, and adolescence
- Heavy alcohol use
- Deficiency of ascorbic acid and/or vitamin B12

Signs and Symptoms of Deficiency

- Atrophy of digestive tract epithelium: reduced absorption of nutrients, diarrhea, anorexia, and weight loss
- Anemia: easy fatigue, weakness, shortness of breath, decreased ability to concentrate

- Reduced production of platelets can increase risk of abnormal bleeding
- Impairments in white blood cell development reduce immune response
- Elevated blood homocysteine with increased risk of atherosclerosis
- Irritability, hostility, forgetfulness, paranoid behavior, depression
- Impaired fetal growth and development, birth defects

Laboratory Measurement of Status

Measure	Values	Comments
Serum folate	Normal levels are 4.5–30 nmol/L.	Reflects recent dietary intake.
Erythrocyte folate	Levels < 312 nmol/L indicate deficiency.	Reflects body folate stores.
Hypersegmentation index of the nuclei of neutrophils	The ratio of neutrophils with ≥ 5 lobes to those with ≤ 4 lobes; values $> 30\%$ indicate deficiency.	Can also result from vitamin B12 deficiency and is not reliable during pregnancy.

Good Dietary Sources

Food	Serving Size	µg
Wheat germ	100 g	270
Kidney beans	100 g	250
Spinach	100 g	134
Broccoli	100 g	105
Calf liver	100 g	108

Recommended Daily Intakes

Prevention of Deficiency			Therapeutic Dose Range
	UK RNI (1991)	USA DRI (1998)	Werbach (1990/99)
Men	200 µg	400 µg	400–75 000 µg
Women*	200 µg	400 µg	400–75 000 µg

* excluding pregnant or lactating women

Preferred Form, Bioavailability, and Dosing

Folic acid	Take between or with meals, preferably with the dose divided throughout the day. Easily destroyed by high heat or temperature.

Toxicity

Hathcock LOAEL (1997)	USA UL (1998)
5000 µg/day	1000 µg/day (synthetic folic acid)

Folic acid appears to be nontoxic even at very high doses. Large doses in people with epilepsy may antagonize the actions of anticonvulsant drugs and provoke increased seizures. Gastrointestinal discomfort and altered sleep patterns have been reported at doses > 10 mg/day. Folate supplementation during vitamin B12 deficiency may partially mask the deficiency of B12 and allow progression of neurological damage. When a folate deficiency is suspected, vitamin B12 status should also be determined. If there is doubt, folate supplementation should be accompanied by vitamin B12 supplementation.

Niacin (Vitamin B3)

Nomenclature

Niacin (vitamin B3) is a generic term used to describe the naturally-occurring compounds niacinamide and nicotinic acid.

Conversions

1 mg of niacin = 60 mg tryptophan
= 1 niacin equivalent (NE)
(60 mg tryptophan can be converted into 1 mg niacin)

Functions

- Biosynthesis of fatty acids and steroids
- Energy production
- Health of the skin and mucus membranes, nervous system, and digestive system
- DNA replication and repair
- Antioxidant
- Blood sugar regulation
- Fat and cholesterol metabolism

Increased Risk of Deficiency

- Low intake of protein containing only small amounts of tryptophan
- Deficiencies of vitamin B6 or riboflavin (vitamin B2)
- Malabsorption (inflammatory bowel disease, other digestive disorders)
- Heavy alcohol use

Signs and Symptoms of Deficiency (Pellagra)

- Red, fissured, scaly, hardened patches on the skin in areas exposed to sunlight, such as elbows, knees, backs of the neck and hands, and forearms
- Inflamed, painful swollen tongue, fissures on lips
- Diminished digestive secretions, loss of appetite, bloating, flatulence, vomiting, and diarrhea
- Anxiety, apprehension, fatigue, irritability, headache, insomnia, emotional instability, confusion, and disorientation
- Hallucinations, paranoia, severe depression

Laboratory Measurement of Status

Measure	Values	Comments
Urinary 1-N-methyl-nicotinamide (NMN) and 2-N-pyridone (2-N-P).	Deficiency is indicated by excretion of < 0.8 mg NMN/day and/or < 1.0 mg 2-N-P/day.	Excretion of these major niacin metabolites are good indexes of niacin status.
Erythrocyte nicotinamide adenine nucleotide (NAD)	A ratio of RBC NAD to RBC nicotinamide nucleotide phosphate (NADP) < 1.0 may indicate deficiency.	A sensitive indicator of status.

Good Dietary Sources

Food	Serving Size	mg NEs
Calf liver	100 g	14
Peanuts	100 g	14
Tuna	100 g	10.5
Chicken, breast	100 g	10.5
Halibut	100 g	5.9

Recommended Daily Intakes

Prevention of Deficiency			Therapeutic Dose Range
	UK RNI (1991)	USA DRI (1998)	Werbach (1990/99)
Men	16–17 mg	16 mg	100–4500 mg
Women*	12–13 mg	14 mg	100–4500 mg

*excluding pregnant or lactating women

Preferred Form, Bioavailability, and Dosing

Niacinamide or nicotinic acid	Take with meals, preferably with the dose divided throughout the day. Niacin is stable and can withstand heating and prolonged storage. The side effects of high doses of nicotinic acid are reduced if taken on a full stomach.

Toxicity

Hathcock LOAEL (1997)	USA UL (1998)
500 mg (niacin); 1000 mg (niacinamide) [half these levels for sustained release forms]	35 mg/day

Large doses (>500 mg) of nicotinic acid (but not niacinamide) may cause dilation of capillaries and produce tingling and flushing of the skin. At doses >2500 mg/day, niacin may cause hypotension and dizziness, increased uric acid in the blood, liver dysfunction, increased risk of peptic ulcer, and increased blood sugar. It should be used with caution in persons with gout, diabetes, and liver disease. With chronic use, these side effects usually lessen in severity and are reversible when the nicotinic acid is discontinued. Sustained-release forms of nicotinic acid are associated with increased risk of adverse side effects compared to short-acting forms.

Pantothenic Acid

Functions

- Energy production
- Synthesis of fatty acids, cholesterol, steroid hormones, and vitamins A and D
- Protein and amino acid synthesis
- Formation of the acetylcholine

Increased Risk of Deficiency

- Chronic illness
- Heavy alcohol use
- Strenuous diets for weight loss

Signs and Symptoms of Deficiency

- Vomiting and stomach pain
- Fatigue, headache, insomnia
- Depression
- Numbness and burning sensation in lower legs and feet
- Arthralgias and myalgias
- Anemia

- Fading of hair color
- Reduced immunity: impairment in antibody response

Laboratory Measurement of Status

Measure	Values
Whole blood pantothenic acid	Levels < 1.6 µmol/L indicate deficiency.
Urinary pantothenic acid	A reliable indicator; excretion of < 1 mg/day indicates deficiency.

Good Dietary Sources

Food	Serving Size	mg
Calf liver	100 g	7.9
Peanuts	100 g	2.6
Peas	100 g	2.1
Soybeans	100 g	1.9
Brown rice	100 g	1.7

Recommended Daily Intakes

Prevention of Deficiency			Therapeutic Dose Range
	UK RNI (1991)	USA DRI (1998)	Werbach (1990/99)
Men	3–7 mg	5 mg	50–1000 mg
Women*	3–7 mg	5 mg	50–1000 mg

* excluding pregnant or lactating women

Preferred Form, Bioavailability, and Dosing

Calcium pantothenate or panthenol	Take between or with meals, preferably with the dose divided throughout the day.

Toxicity

Hathcock LOAEL (1997)	USA UL (1998)
None established	None established

High doses may cause mild diarrhea, but calcium pantothenate appears to be nontoxic even at doses of 10 g/day for several months.

Riboflavin (Vitamin B2)

Functions

- Energy production
- Antioxidant (cofactor of glutathione reductase)

Increased Risk of Deficiency

- Periods of rapid growth: childhood and adolescence, pregnancy and lactation
- Malabsorption (gastrointestinal and biliary obstructions, chronic diarrhea, infectious enteritis)
- Medications: thyroxine, oral contraceptives, phenothiazines, barbiturates, antibiotics
- Heavy alcohol use
- Chronic illness, fever, and cancer

Signs and Symptoms of Deficiency

- Reddened, scaly, greasy, painful, and itchy patches on the skin (especially around the nose, mouth, ears, and the labia majora in females and the scrotum in men)
- Painful fissures and cracks at the angles of the mouth (angular stomatitis) and on the lips (cheilosis). Smooth, purplish-colored tongue, sore throat
- Redness, burning, and excessive tearing of the eyes, light sensitivity
- Anemia with decreased production of red blood cells
- Lethargy, depression, personality changes
- May increase risk of developing cataract
- Symptoms of vitamin B6 and niacin (vitamin B3) deficiency (decreased activation of vitamin B6 and reduced conversion of tryptophan to niacin)

Laboratory Measurement of Status

Measure	Values	Comments
Erythrocyte riboflavin	Levels below 15 μg/dL cells indicate deficiency.	Not a sensitive index.
Urinary riboflavin	Excretion < 100 μg/day indicates deficiency.	
Erythrocyte glutathione reductase (a riboflavin-dependent enzyme) and its stimulation by addition of flavin adenine dinucleotide (FAD)	Expressed as an activity ratio: > 1.2 indicates deficiency.	A reliable indicator of status.

Good Dietary Sources

Food	Serving Size	mg
Calf liver	50 g	1.1
Mushrooms	100 g	0.45
Brewer's yeast	10 g	0.4
Spinach	100 g	0.2
Yogurt	100 g	0.18

Riboflavin (vitamin B3) from animal sources appears to be better absorbed than that from plant sources.

Recommended Daily Intakes

Prevention of Deficiency			Therapeutic Dose Range
	UK RNI (1991)	USA DRI (1998)	Werbach (1990/99)
Men	1.3 mg	1.3 mg	10–400 mg
Women*	1.1 mg	1.1 mg	10–400 mg

* excluding pregnant or lactating women

Preferred Form, Bioavailability, and Dosing

Riboflavin (vitamin B2)	Take between or with meals, preferably with the dose divided throughout the day. Although stable to heat, exposure to light will destroy riboflavin.

Toxicity

Hathcock LOAEL (1997)	USA UL (1998)
None established	None established

There are no reports of toxicity associated with riboflavin (vitamin B2) supplementation. Large doses of riboflavin will color the urine dark yellow.

Thiamin (Vitamin B1)

Nomenclature

Formerly termed aneurine

Functions

- Energy metabolism
- Nerve transmission in the brain and peripheral nerves
- Neurotransmitter metabolism (acetylcholine and serotonin)
- Synthesis of collagen and other proteins

Increased Risk of Deficiency

- Heavy alcohol consumption
- Diets that emphasize refined carbohydrates and processed foods
- Older age groups
- High coffee and black tea intake
- Folate deficiency (impairs absorption of thiamin)
- Strenuous physical exertion
- Fever, stress, burns, hyperthyroidism, liver disease
- Periods of rapid growth: pregnancy and lactation, adolescence
- Oral contraceptive use

Signs and Symptoms of Deficiency

- Impaired sensation and reflexes
- Staggering gait, poor balance
- Mental confusion, defects in learning and memory, frequent headache, insomnia
- Personality changes (depression, irritability)
- Muscle tenderness (especially in the calf muscles) and weakness
- Cardiomyopathy, irregular heart beat, shortness of breath, anemia
- Impaired energy production and fatigue
- Impaired protein (collagen) synthesis: poor wound healing
- Diminished antibody response to infection
- Loss of appetite, constipation

Laboratory Measurement of Status

Measure	Values
Whole blood thiamin	Levels < 70 nmol/L indicate deficiency.
Activity of erythrocyte transketolase (ETKA) and its stimulation after addition of thiamin pyrophosphatase (TTP)	Deficiency is indicated by low ETKA (< 5 U/mmol hemoglobin) and > 16 % increase after addition of TTP.

Good Dietary Sources

Food	Serving Size	mg
Brewer's yeast	10 g	1.2
Pork chop	100 g	0.85
Ham	100 g	0.80
Oatmeal	100 g	0.65
Sunflower seeds	30 g	0.6

Recommended Daily Intakes

Prevention of Deficiency			Therapeutic Dose Range
	UK RNI (1991)	USA DRI (1998)	Werbach (1990/99)
Men	0.9–1 mg	1.2 mg	10–1500 mg
Women*	0.8 mg	1.1 mg	10–1500 mg

* excluding pregnant or lactating women

Preferred Form, Bioavailability, and Dosing

Thiamin hydrochloride	Take between or with meals, preferably with the dose divided throughout the day. Thiamin antagonists (thiaminases) in coffee, black tea, raw fish, and certain vegetables can destroy thiamin in foods and/or supplements. Alcohol also reduces the bioavailability of thiamin.

Toxicity

Hathcock LOAEL (1997)	USA UL (1998)
None established	None established

Thiamin is virtually nontoxic. Doses >200 mg may cause drowsiness in some people. Rare, but severe, allergic reactions have been reported when thiamin is given by injection.

Vitamin A (and the Carotenoids)

Nomenclature

Vitamin A is a generic term used for compounds that exhibit the biological activity of retinol. Retinoids include retinol, retinal, retinaldehyde, and retinyl esters, as well as synthetic analogs (e.g., tretinoin) that may or may not have retinol-like activity.

Conversions

1000 retinol equivalents (RE) =	1 mg retinol
	6 mg beta-carotene
	12 mg other carotenoids
	3330 International Units (IU) vitamin A

Functions

- In the retina, transformation of light energy into the nerve impulses the brain perceives as vision
- Proper growth and development of the skin and mucus membranes
- Antibody production by white blood cells and activity of T cells
- Steroid hormone synthesis, including production of corticosteroids, androgens, and estrogens
- Sperm count and motility in males
- Growth and development during childhood and adolescence
- Iron transport and erythrocyte production
- Myelin synthesis in the nervous system
- Bone growth and repair

Increased Risk of Deficiency

- Childhood and adolescence
- Stress, infection, or surgery
- Fat malabsorption
- Newborns (particularly premature infants)
- Medications: cholesterol-lowering drugs, laxatives, barbiturates
- Diabetes and hypothyroidism (conversion of carotenes to vitamin A is impaired)
- Heavy alcohol consumption
- Cigarette smoking
- Exposure to air pollution, toxic metals (cadmium)

Signs and Symptoms of Deficiency

- Dryness, itching, and redness of the conjunctiva
- Inability to adapt to and see in dim light (night blindness)
- Dry, rough, itchy skin with rash
- Dry, brittle hair and nails
- Loss of sense of smell, taste, and appetite
- Fatigue
- Anemia

- Poor growth
- Increased vulnerability to infections
- Increased risk of cancer of the throat, lung, bladder, cervix, prostate, esophagus, stomach, and colon
- Impaired reproduction and fertility
- Increased risk of kidney stones

Laboratory Measurement of Status

Measure	Values	Comments
Plasma retinol	Levels $< 1.05\ \mu mol/L$ indicate deficiency.	Plasma retinol levels are maintained at the expense of liver vitamin A. Thus, plasma retinol levels begin to fall only when vitamin A deficiency is severe.
Vitamin A content of the liver by biopsy	Levels $< 0.07\ \mu mol/g$ indicate deficiency.	An accurate measure of body stores.
Plasma beta-carotene	Normal levels are 0.3–0.6 μmol/L.	
Serum total carotenoids	Levels $< 50\ \mu mol/L$ indicate poor status.	

Good Dietary Sources

Rich sources of preformed vitamin A (retinol)

Food	Serving size	μg
Beef liver	100 g	9100
Cod liver oil	10 g	2550
Egg	1, whole	110
Cheddar cheese	30 g	95
Whole milk	1 dL	30

Rich sources of beta-carotene (and other carotenoids)

Food	Serving Size	μg Vitamin A
Carrot	1, large	810
Sweet potato	1, large	920
Spinach	100 mg	460
Apricots	3	290
Peach	1, large	200

Recommended Daily Intakes

Prevention of Deficiency			Therapeutic Dose Range
	UK RNI (1991)	USA RDA (1989)	Werbach (1990/99)
Men	700 RE	1000 RE	3000–45 000 RE
Women*	600 RE	800 RE	3000–45 000 RE

* excluding pregnant or lactating women. Women planning a pregnancy or who are pregnant should not exceed a daily intake of 2500 RE (from both food and supplements)

Recommendations for daily intake of beta-carotene for prevention are in the range of 2–6 mg. The usual therapeutic dose range is 15–45 mg/day.

Preferred Form, Bioavailability, and Dosing

Vitamin A	Retinol ester (e.g., retinol palmitate)	Take with meals
Beta carotene	Natural source beta-carotene, such as that derived from the sea algae Dunaliella salina, contains both the cis- and trans-isomers of beta-carotene. It also contains small amounts of alpha-carotene, lycopene, cryptoxanthins, and other natural carotenoids. It may have a broader range of activity and is preferable to synthetic beta-carotene (containing only the trans-isomer).	Take with meals

Toxicity

Hathcock LOAEL (1997)
6500 RE/day

High doses of vitamin A can produce severe toxicity (see below), and children are particularly susceptible. Acute toxicity may be induced by single doses of 300 000 RE in adults, 60 000 RE in children, and 30 000 RE in infants. Toxicity is not usually observed in (nonpregnant) adults at doses < 15 000 REs, even when taken for long periods (weeks to months). Vitamin A is a teratogen and doses > 10 000 REs may produce birth defects, even when exposure is as short as one week in early pregnancy. Total daily intake of vitamin A should not exceed 2500 RE during pregnancy. Because their conversion to retinol in the body is tightly regulated, carotenes do not produce vitamin A toxicity. Chronic high intakes (amounts equal to about 1 kg carrots/day) can cause a benign, reversible yellowing of the skin and nails. There is no evidence that beta-carotene, at any dose level, produces birth defects.

Signs and Symptoms of Toxicity

- Bone pain and joint swelling
- Nausea, vomiting, and diarrhea
- Dry skin and lips, hair loss
- Headache and blurred vision
- Enlargement of the liver and spleen
- Hypothyroidism
- Hypercalcemia

Vitamin B6

Nomenclature

Vitamin B6 is the generic term for compounds that exhibit the biological activity of pyridoxine. This includes pyridoxine, pyridoxal, and pyridoxamine, all of which occur in foods.

Functions

- Protein synthesis
- Blood glucose regulation
- Niacin (vitamin B3) formation from tryptophan
- Synthesis of lipids (myelin sheath, polyunsaturated fatty acids [PUFAs] in cell membranes)
- Hemoglobin synthesis and oxygen transport by erythrocytes
- Neurotransmitter synthesis (serotonin, dopamine, and norepinephrine)

Situations of Increased Need

- Rapid growth: childhood and adolescence, pregnancy and lactation
- High alcohol and coffee intake
- High intakes of protein increase the requirement for vitamin B6
- Cigarette smoking
- Older age groups
- Oral contraceptives
- Chronic diseases (asthma, heart disease, diabetes, kidney failure, rheumatoid arthritis)
- Chronic digestive disorders (diarrhea, liver disease, irritable bowel syndrome)

Signs and Symptoms of Deficiency

- Reddened, scaly, greasy, painful, and itchy patches on the skin (especially around the nose, mouth, ears, and the genital area)
- Painful fissures and cracks at the angles of the mouth and on the lips. Smooth, purplish-colored, and painful tongue. Swollen and sore throat
- Anemia
- Decreased leukocyte function, reduced antibody production
- Abnormal brain wave patterns, muscle twitching, convulsions
- Depression, irritability, anxiety, confusion, headache, insomnia
- Burning, tingling in hands and feet, difficulty walking
- May increase blood total cholesterol and LDL-cholesterol, lower HDL-cholesterol
- May increase risk of calcium oxalate kidney stones

Laboratory Measurement of Status

Measure	Values	Comments
Plasma pyridoxal-5-phosphate (PLP)	Levels < 30 nmol/L indicate deficiency.	The active form of vitamin B6.
Plasma total vitamin B6	Levels < 40 nmol/L indicate deficiency.	
Urinary 4-pyridoxic acid	Levels < 3.0 μmol/day indicate deficiency.	The major urinary metabolite.
Erythrocyte alanine transaminase index	A ratio > 1.25 indicates deficiency.	Activity of this PLP-dependent enzyme is measured before and after addition of PLP.
Tryptophan load test	Urinary xanthenuric acid (XA) excretion > 65 μmol/L indicates deficiency.	Because tryptophan catabolism is PLP-dependent, a 2 g oral tryptophan load is given and XA is measured.

Good Dietary Sources

Food	Serving Size	mg
Calf liver	100 g	0.9
Potatoes	1, average size	0.7
Banana	1, average size	0.6
Lentils	100 g	0.6
Spinach	100 g	0.2

Recommended Daily Intakes

Prevention of Deficiency			Therapeutic Dose Range
	UK RNI (1991)	USA DRI (1998)	Werbach (1990/99)
Men	1.4 mg	1.3–1.7 mg	10–1500 mg
Women*	1.2 mg	1.3–1.5 mg	10–1500 mg

* excluding pregnant or lactating women

Preferred Form, Bioavailability, and Dosing

Pyridoxine hydrochloride is generally preferable to PLP, because it moves more easily through cell membranes and can cross the blood–brain barrier. However, in conditions that impair conversion of pyridoxine hydrochloride to PLP, such as liver disease and zinc or magnesium deficiency, PLP may be preferable.	Take between or with meals, preferably with the dose divided throughout the day. People who have altered sleep patterns when taking vitamin B6 should take most of their daily dose in the morning. Vitamin B6 is sensitive to light and acid conditions.

Toxicity

Hathcock LOAEL (1997)	USA UL (1998)
500 mg/day	100 mg/day

Long-term use of very high doses of vitamin B6 (>1000 mg/day) may cause a peripheral neuropathy characterized by loss of reflexes and numbness and tingling in the hands and feet. This is thought to occur when the liver's capacity to convert vitamin B6 to PLP is exceeded. For this reason, when very high doses are used in therapy, supplements of PLP may be preferred to vitamin B6, as PLP may be associated with less toxicity. Doses of vitamin B6 <500 mg/day, or use of higher doses for short periods (days to weeks) appear to be nontoxic in healthy persons. Very high doses of vitamin B6 may cause breast tenderness or exacerbation of acne, and when given during lactation, may reduce milk production.

Vitamin B12

Nomenclature

Vitamin B12 is the generic term for compounds (cobalamins) that exhibit the biological activity of cyanocobalamin. Hydroxycobalamin and cyanocobalamin are synthetic forms of vitamin B12. The two forms of vitamin B12 naturally occurring in foods are methylcobalamin and 5-deoxyadenosylcobalamin.

Functions

- Activation of folate to its active form (tetrahydrofolate, THF)
- Conversion of homocysteine to methionine
- Fat metabolism
- Synthesis of DNA
- Synthesis of myelin
- Antioxidant (maintains reduced glutathione)

Increased Risk of Deficiency

- Older age groups
- Pernicious anemia
- Atrophic gastritis
- Pregnancy and lactation
- Liver disease
- Intestinal diseases: pancreatic disease, Crohn disease, chronic diarrhea (such as in AIDS)
- Vegan diets
- Heavy alcohol use
- Cigarette smoking
- Medications: paraaminosalicylic acid (PAS), colchicine, neomycin, metformin, cholestyramine

Signs and Symptoms of Deficiency

- Impaired cell replication leads to atrophy and inflammation of mucus membranes in the mouth and entire digestive tract, reduced absorption of nutrients, anorexia, and weight loss
- Anemia (megaloblastic) with weakness, shortness of breath, decreased ability to concentrate
- Reduced production of platelets can increase risk of abnormal bleeding
- Impairments in white blood cell development reduce immune responses
- Irritability, hostility, forgetfulness, confusion, poor memory, agitation, psychosis (with delusions, hallucinations, and/or paranoid behavior), depression
- Numbness and tingling in hands and feet, sensory loss, unsteady movements, poor muscular coordination, unstable gait

Laboratory Measurement of Status

Measure	Values	Comments
Serum vitamin B12	Levels < 150 pmol/L indicate clear deficiency.	Levels may be normal even when anemia or neurological symptoms due to vitamin B12 deficiency are present.
Urinary methylmalonic acid	Levels > 5 µg/mg creatinine indicate deficiency.	A sensitive index of status.
Hypersegmentation index of the nuclei of neutrophils	The ratio of neutrophils with ≥ 5 lobes to those with ≤ 4 lobes; values > 30 % indicate deficiency.	Can also result from folate deficiency and is not reliable during pregnancy.

Good Dietary Sources

Food	Serving Size	µg
Calf liver	100 g	60
Mussels	100 g	8
Salmon	100 g	3
Beef, filet	100 g	2
Egg	1, average size	1

Plant foods, unless they are enriched with the vitamin, contain no vitamin B12. Although colonic bacteria synthesize small amounts of vitamin B12-like compounds, these do not contribute to nutritional needs.

Recommended Daily Intakes

Prevention of Deficiency			Therapeutic Dose Range
	UK RNI (1991)	USA DRI (1998)	Werbach (1990/99)
Men	1 µg	2.4 µg	10–2000 µg
Women*	1 µg	2.4 µg	10–2000 µg

* excluding pregnant or lactating women

Preferred Form, Bioavailability, and Dosing

Hydroxy-cobalamin or adenosyl-cobalamin	Take between or with meals, preferably with the dose divided throughout the day. In older people and those with stomach disorders, intramuscular injection may provide better bioavailability.

Toxicity

Hathcock LOAEL (1997)	USA UL (1998)
None established	None established

There are no reports of toxicity in healthy adults, even at very high oral doses (> 10 mg/day). Intravenous injection is rarely associated with allergic reactions, which can be severe (very likely due to another component of the injected solution and not the vitamin B12).

Vitamin C (Ascorbic Acid)

Nomenclature

Vitamin C is the generic term for compounds that exhibit the biological activity of ascorbic acid. These include L-ascorbic acid and L-dehydroascorbic acid.

Functions

- Antioxidant
- Collagen synthesis
- Carnitine synthesis
- Neurotransmitter synthesis (norepinephrine and serotonin)
- Detoxification and excretion of drugs and chemicals
- Immunocompetence
- Cholesterol breakdown and excretion
- Promotion of iron absorption
- Protects folate and vitamin E from oxidation and maintains these vitamins in their active forms
- Control of blood histamine levels
- Production of epinephrine

Situations of Increased Need

- Increased physical stress (infection, fever, burns, surgery, trauma to soft tissues or bones)
- Chronic illnesses (hyperthyroidism, rheumatoid arthritis, diabetes, chronic kidney failure)
- Heavy alcohol use
- Increased oxidant stress from chemicals, radiation, and heavy metals
- Medications: aspirin, oral contraceptives
- Older age groups
- Rapid growth: childhood, adolescence, pregnancy, and lactation
- Cigarette smoking

Signs and Symptoms of Deficiency (Scurvy)

- Impaired connective tissue synthesis and fragility of blood vessels causes abnormal bleeding: easy bruising, inflamed and bleeding gums, joint stiffness and pain (due to bleeding into joints).
- Buildup of keratin in hair follicles producing roughened „sandpaper skin".
- Impaired wound healing.
- Weakness, lassitude, fatigue (may be due to impaired carnitine synthesis).
- Psychological/neurological symptoms, including depression and personality changes (may be due to impaired neurotransmitter synthesis).
- Impaired immunity with increased risk of infection.
- Diminished antioxidant defenses may increase risk for cancer, heart disease, stroke, cataract.

Laboratory Measurement of Status

Measure	Values	Comments
Plasma ascorbate	Levels < 23 µmol/L indicate deficiency.	
Leukocyte ascorbate	Levels < 114 nmol/10^8 cells (buffy coat) indicate deficiency.	
Urinary ascorbate	Excretion of < 10 mg/day indicates severe deficiency.	An insensitive index of status except in severe deficiency.

Measure	Values	Comments
Ascorbate loading test	Urinary ascorbate is measured after an oral dose of 0.5–2 g over 4 days; excretion of < 60 % of dose indicates tissue ascorbate depletion.	

Good Dietary Sources

Food	Serving Size	mg
Papaya	1, medium	195
Broccoli	100 g	115
Cauliflower	100 g	115
Orange	1, medium	70
Strawberries	100 g	65

Recommended Daily Intakes

Prevention of Deficiency			Therapeutic Dose Range
	UK RNI (1991)	USA DRI (2000)	Werbach (1990/99)
Men	40 mg	90 mg	50 mg–200 g
Women*	40 mg	75 mg	50 mg–200 g

* excluding pregnant or lactating women

Preferred Form, Bioavailability, and Dosing

As ascorbic acid, calcium ascorbate, or sodium ascorbate. Sustained-release forms provide better bioavailability. Buffered forms (salts) are less acidic.	Take between or with meals, preferably with the dose divided throughout the day. Sensitive to heat and oxidation.

Toxicity

Hathcock LOAEL (1997)	USA UL (2000)
None established	2000 mg/day

Several large studies giving 5–10 g of vitamin C daily to healthy humans for several years have demonstrated no adverse effects, other than occasional nausea, loose stools, and diarrhea. Although there have been reports warning of an increased risk of kidney stones with high intakes of vitamin C (oxalate is a metabolite of ascorbic acid), large doses of vitamin C do not increase oxalate excretion into the urine and do not contribute to kidney stones in healthy people. However, in people with a history of kidney stones or kidney disease, doses > 100 mg should be given only under medical supervision. There is no evidence supporting contentions that high doses of vitamin C can cause conditioned scurvy or reduce availability of vitamin B12. High doses of vitamin C may decrease copper absorption. Chewable forms of vitamin C, because of their acidity, can cause erosion of the dental enamel.

Vitamin D

Nomenclature

Vitamin D is the generic term for compounds that exhibit the biological activity of cholecalciferol. These include vitamin D2 (ergocalciferol), vitamin D3 (cholecalciferol), 25-(OH)D3 (calcifediol), 1–25 $(OH)_2D3$ (calcitriol), and dihydrotachysterol

Conversions

1 μg vitamin D = 40 International Units (IU) vitamin D.

Functions

- Calcium absorption and mineral deposition into the skeleton
- Cell growth and development, particularly white blood cells and epithelial cells
- Activity and response of white blood cells against infection

Increased Risk of Deficiency

- Vegetarian diets
- Older age groups
- Inadequate sunlight exposure, northern latitudes, winter season
- Fat malabsorption
- Breast-fed infants
- Chronic kidney disease

Signs and Symptoms of Deficiency

Children

- Delayed growth and development (child begins crawling and walking late)
- Irritability and restlessness
- Rickets: softening of bones, spinal deformities, bowed legs and knock knees, enlargement of the rib–sternum joints
- Delayed tooth eruption and poorly formed tooth enamel
- Impaired immune response with increased risk of infection

Adolescents

- Impaired growth of bones and musculature
- Swelling and pain at the end of long bones, especially at the knee
- Impaired immune response with increased risk of infection

Adults

- Loss of bone mineral from the skeleton, increased risk of osteoporosis and fractures
- Hearing loss and ringing in the ears
- Muscle weakness, particularly around the hip and pelvis
- May increase risk of colorectal and breast cancer
- May increase risk of high blood pressure
- Impaired immune response with increased risk of infection

Laboratory Measurement of Status

Measure	Values	Comments
Plasma 25-(OH) vitamin D	Levels $<$25 nmol/L indicate deficiency.	Reflects body reserves.
Plasma 1–25 $(OH)_2$ vitamin D	Normal levels are 48–100 pmol/L.	Measures current biological activity of the vitamin.

Good Dietary Sources

Food	Serving Size	µg
Salmon	100 g	16
Tuna	100 g	5
Eggs	1, medium	1
Calf liver	100 mg	1
Emmental cheese	30 mg	0.33

In children and young adults, sunlight exposure of the face, arms, and hands for 10–15 minutes is roughly equivalent to ingestion of 5 µg vitamin D.

Recommended Daily Intakes

Prevention of Deficiency			Therapeutic Dose Range
	UK RNI (1991)	USA DRI (1997)	Werbach (1990/99)
Men	0–10 µg	5–15 µg	10–40 µg
Women*	0–10 µg	5–15 µg	10–40 µg

* excluding pregnant or lactating women

Preferred Form, Bioavailability, and Dosing

Cholecalciferol (vitamin D3) is more potent and bioavailable than ergocalciferol (vitamin D2).	Take with meals

Toxicity

Hathcock LOAEL (1997)	USA UL (1998)
50 µg/day	50 µg/day

There is a wide range of susceptibility to the toxicity of vitamin D. The margin of safety, particularly in children, is narrow. In children, intakes of > 100 µg/day may cause hypercalcemia and doses > 45 µg/day may slow growth. In adults, chronic doses > 250 µg/day for 6 months may result in toxicity; chronic intakes > 1000 µg/day can cause renal calcification.

Vitamin E

Nomenclature

Vitamin E is the generic term for tocopherol and tocotrienol compounds that exhibit the biological activity of alpha-tocopherol. The relative biological activity of the common tocopherols are: alpha-tocopherol, 100; beta-tocopherol, 50; gamma-tocopherol, 10–30; and delta-tocopherol, 1.

Conversions

1 tocopherol equivalent (TE)	=	1 mg natural d-alpha tocopherol
	=	0.67 International Units (IU) vitamin E
	=	0.67 mg synthetic dl-alpha tocopherol

Functions

- Antioxidant
- Antithrombotic

Increased Risk of Deficiency

- Consumption of only processed, refined cereals
- High intakes of polyunsturated fatty acids (PUFAs)
- Urban environments, air and water pollution
- Selenium deficiency
- Fat malabsorption
- Newborn infants, and particularly premature infants
- Repeated strenuous exercise

Signs and Symptoms of Deficiency

- Decreased membrane integrity of red blood cells produces hemolysis and anemia
- Degeneration of nerve cells
- Atrophy and weakness in skeletal and smooth muscles
- Atrophy of the reproductive organs and infertility
- May increase risk of cancer, atherosclerosis, arthritis, and cataract

Laboratory Measurement of Status

Measure	Values	Comments
Plasma vitamin E	Levels < 11.6 μmol/L indicate deficiency.	
Plasma alpha-tocopherol (μmol/L)/ plasma cholesterol (mmol/L)	Ratio < 2.2 indicates deficiency	The vitamin E level in the blood is directly correlated with the blood lipid level. Therefore, to accurately measure vitamin E status, the ratio of vitamin E/total cholesterol is used.
Plasma alpha-tocopherol	Levels < 10 μmol/L generally indicate deficiency.	Normally, > 90 % of total vitamin E is alpha-tocopherol.

Good Dietary Sources

Food	Serving Size	mg
Sunflower seeds	100 g	21
Wheat germ	100 g	12
Sweet potatoes	1, average size	7
Safflower oil	10 g	3.5
Shrimp	100 g	3.5

Recommended Daily Intakes

Prevention of Deficiency			Therapeutic Dose Range
	UK RNI (1991)	USA DRI (2000)	Werbach (1990/99)
Men	> 4 mg	15 mg	100–2500 mg
Women*	> 3 mg	15 mg	100–2500 mg

* excluding pregnant or lactating women

Preferred Form, Bioavailability, and Dosing

Natural vitamin E (d-alpha tocopherol) is the preferred form. It is 50–100 % more bioavailable and more potent than synthetic vitamin E (dl-alpha-tocopherol).	Take with meals. Sensitive to heat and oxidation.

Toxicity

Hathcock LOAEL (1997)	USA UL (2000)
None established	1000 mg/day

At doses of 400–800 mg/day in healthy persons, vitamin E is nontoxic. Daily doses of 1600–3200 mg have been used for prolonged periods without significant side effects. People taking anticoagulant drugs should be cautious with high doses: vitamin E may enhance the effects of anticoagulants and decrease levels of vitamin K–dependent clotting factors. People with diabetes should be cautious when starting to take high doses: vitamin E may enhance the action of insulin and, rarely, produce hypoglycemia.

Vitamin K

Nomenclature

Vitamin K is the generic term for a family of compounds that exhibit the biological activity of phytomenadione. The form found in plant foods is termed phytomenadione or phylloquinone (vitamin K1). The forms synthesized by bacteria are menaquinones (vitamin K2). The parent compound is known as menadione (vitamin K3); it is not a naturally-occurring form and is not used in humans.

Functions

- Hepatic synthesis of coagulation proteins (prothrombin, VII, IX, X, proteins C, S, Z)
- Production of structural and regulatory proteins in bone (e.g., osteocalcin)

Increased Risk of Deficiency

- Liver disease
- Heavy alcohol use
- Medications: broad-spectrum antibiotics, cholestyramine, coumarin
- Fat malabsorption
- Newborn infants who are exclusively breast-fed

Signs and Symptoms of Deficiency

- Prolonged bleeding, small amounts of blood in the stool, easy bruising
- Impaired bone remodeling and mineralization

Laboratory Measurement of Status

Measure	Values	Comments
Plasma vitamin K	Normal levels are 0.4–5.0 nmol/L.	
Prothrombin time and/or clotting factors (X, IX, VII, and protein C).	Normal prothrombin time is 11–14 seconds. Normal values for clotting factors are 100% or 1.0 unit/mL.	Because of vitamin K's central role in blood coagulation, status is measured by indexes of blood clotting. Deficiency results in prolongation of the prothrombin time (PT) and reduced function of vitamin K-dependent clotting factors.

Good Dietary Sources

Food	Serving Size	μg
Spinach	100 g	415
Broccoli	100 g	175
Green cabbage	100 g	125
Beef liver	100 g	92
Tea, green	10 g	71

Synthesis of vitamin K by colonic bacteria can contribute significantly to daily requirements, in some individuals supplying up to half the daily requirement.

Recommended Daily Intakes

Prevention of Deficiency			Therapeutic Dose Range
	UK RNI (1991)	USA RDA (1989)	Werbach (1990/99)
Men	1 μg/kg body weight	80 μg	30–100 μg
Women*	1 μg/kg body weight	65 μg	30–100 μg

* excluding pregnant or lactating women

Preferred Form, Bioavailability, and Dosing

Vitamin K1 (phylloquinone)	Take with meals

Toxicity

Hathcock LOAEL (1997)
None established

Oral ingestion of natural forms of vitamin K is not associated with toxicity, even at doses as high as 4000 μg/day. Menadione, used in the past as a infant supplement, is toxic even at low doses, causing anemia and jaundice. It is no longer used as a therapeutic form of vitamin K.

The Minerals and Trace Elements

Calcium

Functions

- Main structural component of the skeleton and teeth
- Blood clotting
- Intracellular messenger triggering contraction of muscle fibers
- Nerve transmission

Increased Risk of Deficiency

- Older age groups
- Menopause
- Diets containing large amounts of protein, phosphorus, sodium, alcohol, and caffeine (all increase urinary calcium losses)
- Medications: antacids, laxatives, and steroids
- Atrophic gastritis
- Fat malabsorption (fats bind calcium, reducing absorption)
- Vitamin D deficiency

Signs and Symptoms of Deficiency

- Poor bone mineralization, osteoporosis
- Muscle cramping and spasm
- Increased irritability of nerve cells
- Abnormal blood clotting and increased bleeding after trauma

Laboratory Measurement of Status

Measure	Values	Comments
Serum calcium	Normal levels are 2.2–2.6 mmol/L.	A poor indicator of status, as $<1\%$ of body calcium is in serum and the serum level is under tight physiological control.

Measure	Values	Comments
Ionized (unbound) serum calcium	Normal levels are 1.17–1.29 mmol/L.	Low levels may indicate negative calcium balance.
Urinary calcium	Normal levels are approximately 200–300 mg/day for men, 150–250 mg/day for women.	

Good Dietary Sources

Food	Serving Size	mg
Cheese	100 g	830
Sardines (with bones)	100 g	354
Soybeans, dry	100 g	260
Cabbage	100 g	212
Yogurt	180 g	205

Recommended Daily Intakes

Prevention of Deficiency			Therapeutic Dose Range
	UK RNI (1991)	USA DRI (1997)	Werbach (1990/99)
Men	700 mg	1000–1200 mg	1000–3000 mg
Women*	700 mg	1000–1200 mg	1000–3000 mg

* excluding pregnant or lactating women

Preferred Forms, Bioavailability, and Dosing

Organically bound calcium (as gluconate, aspartate, citrate, or chelated forms) is generally more bioavailable than inorganic forms (carbonate, phosphate, sulfate), particularly in people with insufficient gastric acid and in many older adults.	Take with meals, preferably with the dose divided throughout the day.

Toxicity

Hathcock LOAEL (1997)	USA UL (1997)
2500 mg/day	2500 mg/day

In healthy adults, oral intakes of calcium up to 2 g/day do not appear to have significant side effects or toxicity. People with hyperparathyroidism and people who have a tendency to form calcium oxalate kidney stones should avoid high intakes of calcium. However, among the general population, high intakes of calcium do not appear to increase the risk of kidney stones.

Chromium

Functions

- Potentiates the action of insulin: improves glucose tolerance; increases uptake of amino acids into muscle, heart, and liver; enhances protein synthesis
- Regulation of blood lipids: decreases total cholesterol and LDL-cholesterol, and increases HDL-cholesterol

Increased Risk of Deficiency

- Diets high in fat, sugars, and refined carbohydrates
- Increased stress: strenuous exercise, physical activity, infection, trauma, or illness
- Pregnancy
- Older age groups

Signs and Symptoms of Deficiency

- Impaired glucose tolerance and reduced insulin action
- Weight loss
- Elevated cholesterol and triglyceride levels in blood
- Peripheral neuropathy

Laboratory Measurement of Status

Measure	Values	Comments
Serum chromium	< 2.0 nmol/L may indicate deficiency.	A relatively insensitive indicator of tissue stores.
Whole blood chromium	Normal range is 14–185 nmol/L.	
Urinary chromium	Normal range is approximately 3–4 nmol/L; > 38 nmol indicates toxicity.	Of limited value in assessing status due to the very low concentrations involved and the fact that they often do not respond to chromium supplementation. However, they can be used to measure overexposure to chromium.

Good Dietary Sources

Food	Serving Size	μg
Lentils	100 g	70
Whole wheat bread	100 g	49
Molasses	30 g	36
Chicken	100 g	26
Brewer's yeast	10 g	20

Recommended Daily Intakes

Prevention of Deficiency			Therapeutic Dose Range
	UK Safe Intake Level (1991)	USA RDA (1989)	Werbach (1990/99)
Men	25 μg	50–200 μg	200–3000 μg
Women	25 μg	50–200 μg	200–3000 μg

Preferred Forms, Bioavailability, and Dosing

Organic forms of chromium (high chromium yeast, chromium-glucose tolerance factor (GTF), chromium aspartate, picolinate, and nicotinate) are preferable. Chromium chloride is very poorly absorbed (<1 %).	Chromium supplements should be taken between meals, preferably with the dose divided throughout the day.

Toxicity

Hathcock LOAEL (1997)
None established

Chronic daily intake of trivalent chromium (Cr^{+3}) and chromium in brewer's yeast in the range of 100–300 μg is considered generally safe. Supplementation of up to 1000 μg of chromium picolinate for several months in adults has produced no adverse effects. Heavy chronic exposure to airborne hexavalent chromium (Cr^{+6}), produced in metalworking industries, can produce dermatitis and increase the risk of lung cancer.

Copper

Functions

- Energy production in mitochondria
- Mobilization and transfer of iron from storage sites to the bone marrow
- Synthesis of collagen and elastin in connective tissue
- Antioxidant (as zinc/copper superoxide dismutase [Zn/Cu SOD] and ceruloplasmin)
- Synthesis of melanin in the skin
- Synthesis of epinephrine and norepinephrine in the adrenal and nervous system
- Breakdown of serotonin, histamine, and dopamine

Increased Risk of Deficiency

- High intakes of supplemental iron, molybdenum, or zinc
- Infants who are fed only cow's milk (milk is very low in copper)
- Prolonged use of antacids
- Gastrointestinal disorders: chronic diarrhea, inflammatory bowel disease
- Increased oxidative stress (cigarette smoking, air pollution, rheumatoid arthritis)

Signs and Symptoms of Deficiency

- Anemia accompanied by leukopenia and neutropenia
- Increased vulnerability to oxidative damage
- Hypercholesterolemia, hypertriglyceridemia, and glucose intolerance
- May increase fragility of blood vessel walls and increase risk of aneurysm
- May reduce immune responses and impair activation of T cells
- Abnormal skeletal growth, osteoporosis
- Changes and loss of hair and skin pigmentation, and vitiligo
- Weakness and fatigue

Laboratory Measurement of Status

Measure	Values	Comments
Erythrocyte Cu/Zn superoxide dismutase	Normal values are 0.47 ± 0.067 mg/g Hb.	A good index of copper status.
Serum copper	Levels < 12 μmol/L indicate deficiency.	Can be used to detect copper deficiency, but is elevated by a variety of conditions and can vary independently of body copper.
Plasma ceruloplasmin	Normal levels are 0.1–0.5 g/L.	> 90 % of blood copper is bound to ceruloplasmin. Because ceruloplasmin is an acute-phase protein it can vary independently of body copper.
Urinary copper	Normal levels are 0.47–0.94 μmol/day.	

Good Dietary Sources

Food	Serving Size	mg
Liver (calf)	100 g	3.5–5.5
Certain ports and sherry	50 mL	3–10
Oysters	100 g	2.5
Lentils, chick peas, kidney beans	100 g	0.7–0.8
Sunflower seeds	25 g	0.7

Recommended Daily Intakes

Prevention of Deficiency			Therapeutic Dose Range
	UK RNI (1991)	USA RDA (1989)	Werbach (1990/99)
Men	1.2 mg	1.5–3 mg	2–10 mg
Women	1.2 mg	1.5–3 mg	2–10 mg

Preferred Forms, Bioavailability, and Dosing

Although copper sulfate is the most common supplemental form, organically-bound forms of copper (orotate, chelates) may be more bioavailable.	Copper supplements should be taken between meals, preferably with the dose divided throughout the day.

Toxicity

Hathcock LOAEL (1997)
None established

Copper is generally well-tolerated and appears safe at doses of up to 5 mg/day in healthy adults. In adults, doses of > 7 mg/day may produce abdominal pain, nausea, vomiting, and diarrhea, and higher doses can cause liver damage.

Fluoride

Functions

- Increased resistance of tooth enamel to acid formed by oral bacteria
- Stimulation of osteoblast activity

Signs and Symptoms of Deficiency

- Increased susceptibility to dental caries

Laboratory Measurement of Status

Measure	Values
Whole blood fluoride	Normal levels are 0.1–0.25 mg/L
Plasma fluoride	Normal levels are 4–14 µg/L
Urinary fluoride	Normal levels are 0.3–1.5 mg/day

Good Dietary Sources

Source	Serving Size	mg
Fluoridated water*	1 L	0.7–1.2
Canned sardines (including bones)	100 g	0.2–0.4
Tea (brewed with nonfluoridated water)	100 mL	0.01–0.42
Fluoridated salt	1 g	0.25
Chicken	100 g	0.06–0.1

* natural fluoride levels in water range from 0.01–2 mg/100 mL. Many children obtain additional fluoride by ingesting fluoride-containing toothpastes that usually contain about 1–1.5 mg/g.

Recommended Daily Intakes

Age (years)	USA DRI (1997)
0–0.5	0.01 mg
0.5–1	0.5 mg
1–3	0.7 mg
4–8	1.0 mg
9–13	2.0 mg
14–18	3.0 mg
Adults	3.0–4.0 mg

Recommended fluoride supplement dose (mg/day) at different concentrations of fluoride in drinking water

Age	<0.3 mg/L	0.3–0.6 mg/L	>0.7 mg/L
0–6 months	0	0	0
6 months–3 years	0.25	0	0
3–6 years	0.5	0.25	0
6–16 years	1	0.5	0

Preferred Forms, Bioavailability, and Dosing

As sodium fluoride	At bedtime, after toothbrushing.

Toxicity

Hathcock LOAEL (1997)	USA UL (1997)
4–20 mg/day	10 mg/day

Chronic intakes of up to 5 mg fluoride/day in healthy adults appear to be safe. As intakes rise above this level, toxicity occurs. The first sign is dental fluorosis, in which the excess fluoride interferes with mineralization of the enamel and produces weakened, stained, and pitted enamel. Ingestion of >8–10 mg fluoride/day may produce skeletal deformities, osteoporosis, and osteomalacia, along with secondary hyperparathyroidism and calcification of soft tissues.

Iodine

Function

- Synthesis of thyroid hormones

Increased Risk of Deficiency

- Diets originating from inland and mountainous areas of the world where the soil is deficient in iodine
- Pregnancy and lactation
- Goitrogens in the diet (cassava, millet, *Brassica* vegetables) and industrial pollutants (resorcinol, phthalic acid)

Signs and Symptoms of Deficiency

- In the fetus: increased abortion, stillbirths, and congenital defects (mental retardation, deafness, spasticity)
- In infancy: increased infant mortality, psychomotor and mental impairment, hypothyroidism
- In childhood: goiter, hypothyroidism, impaired mental function and physical growth
- In adulthood: goiter, hypothyroidism, impaired mental function
- The signs and symptoms of hypothyroidism include weight gain, edema, fatigue, lack of energy, a slow heart rate, low blood pressure, hair loss, and dry skin

Laboratory Measurement of Status

Measure	Values	Comments
Urinary iodine	Excretion < 0.78 µmol/day indicates deficiency.	A reliable indicator of status.
Serum total thyroxine (T_4)	Normal range 68–182 nmol/L.	Severe iodine deficiency may cause hypothyroidism.
Serum thyroid-stimulating hormone (TSH)	Values > 4.0 mU/L may indicate iodine deficiency or another cause of thyroid impairment.	

Good Dietary Sources

Food	Serving Size	μg
Mussels, clams, salmon	100 g	200–250
Shrimp, cod	100 g	120–130
Mackerel, tuna, herring, halibut	100 g	50–75
Iodized salt	1 g	15–40

Recommended Daily Intakes

Prevention of Deficiency			Therapeutic Dose Range
	UK RNI (1991)	USA RDA (1989)	Werbach (1990/99)
Men	140 μg	150 μg	100–230 μg
Women*	140 μg	150 μg	100–230 μg

* excluding pregnant or lactating women

Preferred Forms, Bioavailability, and Dosing

Kelp (sea algae) or potassium iodide	Take with or between meals.

Toxicity

Hathcock LOAEL (1997)
None established

Iodide intake at levels of 100–500 μg/day is essentially nontoxic. Although iodide can occasionally precipitate acne in susceptible individuals, high levels of intake (up to 1 mg/day) are well tolerated in most healthy adults. However, very high daily intake (>2 mg/day) may impair thyroid hormone production. Moreover, in people with long-standing iodine deficiency and goiter, abruptly increasing iodine intake may cause hyperthyroidism and, rarely, thyrotoxicosis.

Iron

Functions

- Oxygen transport as hemoglobin in erythrocytes
- Oxygen storage as myoglobin within muscle cells
- Energy production in mitochondrial cytochromes
- Cofactor for multiple enzymes, including the cytochrome P450 system in liver, the antioxidant peroxidases, and catalase
- Production of brain neurotransmitters and thyroid hormone

Increased Risk of Deficiency

- Menstruating women
- Rapid growth: childhood and adolescence, pregnancy
- Infants and young children consuming mainly milk (milk has very little iron)
- Vegetarian diets
- High intake of coffee or black tea with meals
- Atrophic gastritis
- Chronic use of antacids
- Digestive tract losses: hemorrhoids, small ulcers, gastric irritation from aspirin or other nonsteroidal anti-inflammatory drugs, steroid use, or heavy alcohol intake
- Long-distance running and swimming
- Chronic illness (reduces the ability to mobilize iron from stores)
- Deficiencies of vitamin A, vitamin B6, and copper

Signs and Symptoms of Deficiency

- Anemia, pallor, dry skin, poorly-formed, upturned nails, brittle hair
- Easily tired, weakness, lack of energy
- Loss of appetite
- Inability to maintain body warmth when exposed to cold
- Learning difficulties: impaired memory and concentration
- Impaired mental and motor development during childhood
- Inflammation of the oral mucosa
- Increased susceptibility to infection
- Increased uptake and vulnerability to environmental lead and cadmium
- In athletes: reduced performance, early fatigue, increased lactic acid production in muscles, and muscle cramping
- In pregnancy: increased risk of premature birth and of delivering a low-birthweight infant

Laboratory Measurement of Status

Measure	Values	Comments
Serum iron	Normal levels are 9–29 μmol/L.	An insensitive indicator of status, falling only after stores are completely exhausted.
Serum ferritin	Normal levels are 12–200 μg/L.	A good indicator of body stores, but may be increased by inflammation/infection independent of status.
Transferrin saturation	Saturation of < 16 % of available binding sites indicates iron deficiency.	
Serum transferrin receptor	Levels > 8 mg/L indicate deficiency.	Indicates body stores independent of inflammation or infection.

Good Dietary Sources

Food	Serving Size	mg
Liver (pork)	100 g	20
Oysters	100 g	13
Soy flour, millet	100 g	9
Liver (beef, veal)	100 g	7–8
Lentils	100 g	7

The bioavailability of iron from foods varies greatly, ranging from < 2 % in certain high-fiber plant foods, to 15–20 % from meats, to nearly 50 % from human breast milk.

Recommended Daily Intakes

Prevention of Deficiency			Therapeutic Dose Range
	UK RNI (1991)	USA RDA (1989)	Werbach (1990/99)
Men	8.7 mg	10 mg	10–200 mg
Women*	8.7–14.8 mg	15 mg	10–200 mg

* excluding pregnant or lactating women

Preferred Forms, Bioavailability, and Dosing

Ferrous fumarate and iron-EDTA may be more bioavailable then ferrous sulfate, especially in individuals with low gastric acidity. Elemental iron is very poorly absorbed.	Iron supplements should usually be taken between meals. However, gastrointestinal side effects are more common when iron is taken on an empty stomach. If abdominal pain or nausea occur, taking the iron with meals may reduce these side effects. Taking iron together with a vitamin C supplement or vitamin C–rich food will increase bioavailability of the iron 2–3 fold.

Toxicity

Hathcock LOAEL (1997)
100 mg/day

Acute iron poisoning in young children can be fatal. A lethal dose of iron is about 2–2.5 g in a 10 kg child. To treat anemia, iron is often given in high doses of 30–60 mg per day. At this level, particularly on an empty stomach, supplements can cause abdominal pain, nausea, and vomiting. In hereditary hemochromatosis (HH), a common inherited defect in the regulation of iron absorption, the risk of iron overload and chronic toxicity is sharply increased. About 1 in 10 people are heterozygous for this disorder and may be vulnerable to damage from excess iron. Iron is a powerful oxidant and iron overload can do widespread damage. In the liver, it produces chronic inflammation and injury that increases the risk of liver cancer. Iron overload may also increase the risk of coronary heart disease. Screening for HH, by measuring transferrin saturation, can detect the disorder before clinical signs of overload occur.

Magnesium

Functions

- Energy metabolism: oxidation of glucose, fat, and proteins
- Regulation of calcium-triggered contraction of heart and muscle cells
- Vasodilation of the coronary and peripheral arteries
- Nerve depolarization and transmission
- Structure of the bones and teeth

Increased Risk of Deficiency

- Diets emphasizing processed foods, refined grains, and few vegetables
- Strenuous athletic training
- Rapid growth: pregnancy and lactation, childhood and adolescence
- Medications: diuretics (thiazides, furosemide), chemotherapy (cisplatin), steroids, laxatives
- Diabetes and hyperparathyroidism
- Intestinal malabsorption (inflammatory bowel disease, diarrhea, pancreatic disease)
- High intakes of alcohol

Signs and Symptoms of Deficiency

- Muscle cramps and spasm, trembling
- Hypocalcemia and hypokalemia
- Personality changes: depression, irritability, difficulty concentrating
- Anorexia, nausea, and vomiting
- May increase risk of arrythymias
- Increased blood triglycerides and cholesterol
- Sodium and water retention
- Impaired action of vitamin D

Laboratory Measurement of Status

Measure	Values	Comments
Serum magnesium	Normal levels are 0.75–1.05 mmol/L.	An insensitive index of body stores, as levels fall only if deficiency is advanced.
Serum ionized magnesium	Normal levels are 0.5–0.66 mmol/L.	Superior to serum levels, because the portion of blood magnesium that is ionized is not affected by conditions that alter serum proteins.
Leukocyte magnesium	Normal levels are 3.0–4.0±0.09 fmol/cell.	Levels may reflect tissue levels.
Urinary magnesium	Excretion of <1 mmol/day indicates deficiency.	A sensitive measure of status.

Good Dietary Sources

Food	Serving Size	mg
Soy flour	100 g	245
Whole-grain rice, barley	100 g	160
Wheat bran	25 g	145–150
Sunflower seeds	25 g	105
Whole wheat bread	100 g	80–100

Recommended Daily Intakes

Prevention of Deficiency			Therapeutic Dose Range
	UK RNI (1991)	USA DRI (1997)	Werbach (1990/99)
Men	300 mg	420 mg	300–1000 mg
Women*	270–300 mg	320 mg	300–1000 mg

* excluding pregnant or lactating women

Preferred Forms, Bioavailability, and Dosing

Organically-bound forms of magnesium (as orotate, gluconate, aspartate, citrate, or chelated forms) are generally more bioavailable than inorganic forms (e.g., sulfate).	Take with meals, preferably with the dose divided throughout the day.

Toxicity

Hathcock LOAEL (1997)	USA UL (1997)
None established	350 mg/day

In healthy adults, magnesium at doses up to 1 g/day appear to be nontoxic. In people with chronic kidney failure, urinary excretion of magnesium is impaired, and supplements (or magnesium-containing antacids or laxatives) can produce high blood levels with symptoms of nausea, vomiting, low blood pressure, and arrythymias.

Manganese

Functions

- Carbohydrate metabolism and gluconeogenesis
- Insulin synthesis and secretion
- Antioxidant (as Mn-superoxide dismutase)
- Amino acid breakdown and production of urea
- Synthesis of proteoglycans in cartilage and bone
- Enzyme activation, including the breakdown histamine, the regulation of neurotransmitters in the brain, production of prothrombin in blood clotting, and lipid metabolism

Increased Risk of Deficiency

- Diets that emphasize refined carbohydrates, processed foods, and animal products
- Increased oxidant stress from environmental sources
- High alcohol intake
- High-dose iron supplementation

Signs and Symptoms of Deficiency

- Reduction in HDL-cholesterol and total cholesterol in the blood, fatty liver
- Impaired production of bone and cartilage
- Increased vulnerability to oxidative damage
- Dermatitis, reduced hair and nail growth, reddening of hair
- Decreased appetite and weight loss
- Impaired insulin secretion, reduced ability to control blood sugar, glucose intolerance

Laboratory Measurement of Status

Measure	Values	Comments
Whole blood manganese	Normal levels are 72–255 nmol/L.	A valid indicator of status.
Urinary manganese	Normal levels are 10.6 ± 1.9 nmol/day; > 180 nmol/L indicates toxicity.	

Good Dietary Sources

Food	Serving Size	mg
Oatmeal	100 g	5
Soy flour	100 g	4
Whole wheat flour	100 g	3.5
Hazelnuts	50 g	3
Whole wheat bread	100 g	2.5

Recommended Daily Intakes

Prevention of Deficiency			Therapeutic Dose Range
	UK Safe Intake Level (1991)	USA RDA (1989)	Werbach (1990/99)
Men	1.4 mg	2–5 mg	2–190 mg
Women	1.4 mg	2–5 mg	2–190 mg

Preferred Forms, Bioavailability, and Dosing

Organically-bound forms (manganese gluconate, or chelates) generally have greater bioavailability than manganese sulfate.	Take with meals, preferably with the dose divided throughout the day.

Toxicity

Hathcock LOAEL (1997)
None established

Manganese supplements in the range of 2–50 mg per day appear to be safe in healthy adults. Manganese toxicity can occur as a result of exposure to high amounts of environmental manganese (industrial workers) and produces psychosis with hyperirritability and violence, incoordination, dementia, and symptoms similar to Parkinson disease.

Molybdenum

Functions

- Antioxidant (as xanthine oxidase)
- Protection from toxic effects of chemicals and drugs (as molybdenum hydroxylase)
- Transport and storage of iron in tissues
- Metabolism and breakdown of sulfur-containing amino acids (such as cysteine, methionine, taurine, homocysteine), as well as the conversion of sulfite (a toxic compound) to sulfate

Increased Risk of Deficiency

- Consumption of diets high in refined carbohydrates, fats and oils, and meat products
- Exposure to drugs and chemicals
- Increased oxidant stress
- Digestive disorders that produce diarrhea and malabsorption (e.g., Crohn disease)

Signs and Symptoms of Deficiency

- Decreased uric acid production and a reduction in antioxidant protection
- Impaired metabolism of potentially toxic sulfur-containing amino acids (cysteine, methionine, homocysteine) which can produce central nervous system (CNS) disorders
- Increased sensitivity to sulfites in the environment (air pollution) and in the diet (salads, dried fruits, wine)
- Hair loss
- Fatigue
- May increase risk of cancer (particularly cancer of the esophagus)
- May increase risk of kidney stones (xanthine stones)

Laboratory Measurement of Status

Measure	Values
Serum molybdenum	Normal values are 6.0–8.3±2.1 nmol/L.

Good Dietary Sources

Food	Serving Size	µg
Soy flour	100 g	180
Red cabbage	100 g	120
White beans	100 g	100
Potatoes	100 g	5–85
Whole-grain rice	100 g	80

Recommended Daily Intakes

Prevention of Deficiency			Therapeutic Dose Range
	UK Safe Intake Level (1991)	USA RDA (1989)	Werbach (1990/99)
Men	50–400 µg	75–250 µg	100–2000 µg
Women	50–400 µg	75–250 µg	100–2000 µg

Preferred Forms, Bioavailability, and Dosing

Sodium molybdenate	Take with meals, preferably with the dose divided throughout the day.

Toxicity

Hathcock LOAEL (1997)
None established

Molybdenum, at doses <1 mg /day, appears to be nontoxic in healthy adults. At very high doses (10–20 times higher than in normal diets), molybdenum may increase the production of uric acid and precipitate gout.

Potassium

Functions

- Energy production
- Membrane excitability and transport

Situations of Increased Need

- Diarrhea and/or vomiting
- Inflammatory bowel disease or gastroenteritis
- Chronic kidney failure
- Strenuous diets for weight loss
- Metabolic acidosis or alkalosis
- Diuretics (thiazides, furosemide)
- Deficiency of magnesium

Signs and Symptoms of Deficiency

- Fatigue, lethargy
- Muscle weakness
- Delayed gastric emptying
- Constipation
- Decreased blood pressure
- Cardiac arrythmias

Laboratory Measurement of Status

Measure	Values	Comments
Serum potassium	Normal levels are 3.5–5.1 mmol/L.	
Erythrocyte potassium	Normal levels are approximately 100 mmol/L red blood cells (RBCs).	An index of tissue potassium stores.
Urinary potassium	Normal levels are 26–123 mmol/day.	Level varies with dietary intake.

Good Dietary Sources

Food	Serving Size	mg
Soy flour	100 g	1870
White beans	100 g	1310
Lentils	100 g	810
Bananas	200 g	790
Spinach	100 g	635

Recommended Daily Intakes

The minimum daily requirement for potassium in healthy adults is estimated to be 2 g. The average intake among the adult population of the industrialized world is approximately 2–3 g per day. However, recommended daily intakes to reduce risk of high blood pressure, stroke, and heart disease, are higher—in the range of 4–5 g/day.

Preferred Forms, Bioavailability, and Dosing

Potassium citrate is generally better tolerated than potassium chloride.	Take with meals, preferably with the dose divided throughout the day.

Toxicity

Hyperkalemia can produce cardiac arrythmias, weakness and fatigue, nausea, and a fall in blood pressure. In healthy adults, daily intakes >8 g can produce hyperkalemia. In people with kidney and/or heart disease, the daily dose that is toxic is sharply lower.

Selenium

Functions

- Antioxidant (as glutathione peroxidase)
- Immune modulation: regulation of the production of IgG and tumor necrosis factor, enhancement of white blood cell activity
- Activation of thyroid hormone in peripheral tissues

Increased Risk of Deficiency

- Regions where soil selenium levels are low (e.g., Scandinavia, central Europe, New Zealand, and parts of China and Africa)
- Increased oxidative stress: strenuous exercise or physical activity, cigarette smoking, exposure to environmental chemicals, chronic illness (e.g., rheumatoid arthritis)
- Digestive disorders causing malabsorption: pancreatic disorders, cystic fibrosis, and the inflammatory bowel diseases
- HIV disease, AIDS

Signs and Symptoms of Deficiency

- Decreased resistance to oxidative damage
- May increase risk of developing cancer
- Cardiomyopathy and heart failure (Keshan disease)
- May weaken the immune system and increase risk of infection
- Childhood osteoarthritis (Kashin–Beck disease)
- Muscle weakness

Laboratory Measurement of Status

Measure	Values	Comments
Blood glutathione peroxidase activity	Activity <30 E/g hemoglobin indicates deficiency.	A sensitive index of status.
Serum selenium	Normal range is 0.9–1.9 μmol/L.	An index of short-term dietary intake.

Good Dietary Sources

Food	Serving Size	μg
Herring, tuna	100 g	120–140
Sardines	100 g	80–100
Liver (calf)	100 g	50–70
Soybeans	100 g	50–70
Whole wheat bread	100 g	30–60

Recommended Daily Intakes

Prevention of Deficiency			Therapeutic Dose Range
	UK RNI (1991)	USA DRI (2000)	Werbach (1990/99)
Men	75 μg	55 μg	200–1000 μg
Women*	60 μg	55 μg	200–1000 μg

* excluding pregnant or lactating women

Preferred Forms, Bioavailability, and Dosing

Organic forms of selenium (selenomethionine, selenocysteine, selenium-rich yeast, and selenium aspartate) are preferable. Sodium selenite is less bioavailable.	Take with meals, preferably with the dose divided throughout the day.

Toxicity

Hathcock LOAEL (1997)	USA UL (2000)
910 μg/day	400 μg/day

Daily intakes of up to 400–500 μg/day appear to be safe in healthy adults. Chronic intakes > 900 μg/day are associated with nausea, vomiting, hair loss, nail changes, fatigue, and peripheral neuropathy.

Zinc

Functions

- Cofactor in multiple enzymes: RNA polymerases (synthesis of new proteins); alcohol dehydrogenase; DNA synthesis; neurotransmitter metabolism; metabolism of a variety of hormones (growth hormone, thyroid hormone, insulin, and the sex hormones)
- Cell growth and differentiation
- Production and regulation of the cellular and humoral immune response
- Cytoprotective against organic toxins, heavy metals, radiation, and endotoxins produced by pathogenic bacteria
- Antioxidant (as part of copper/zinc superoxide dismutase)

Increased Risk of Deficiency

- Rapid growth: childhood and adolescence, pregnancy and lactation
- Vegetarian and semivegetarian diets
- Chronic dieting for weight loss
- Digestive disorders: pancreatic insufficiency, inflammatory bowel diseases, diarrhea
- Acrodermatitis enteropathica
- High-dose calcium supplements
- Heavy consumption of alcohol
- Liver and kidney disease, diabetes
- Chronic infection or inflammatory disease (such as rheumatoid arthritis)

Signs and Symptoms of Deficiency

- Dermatitis, inflammatory acne, reduced wound healing, hair loss
- Reduced sense of smell, taste (often accompanied by anorexia)
- Slow growth, stunting, delayed sexual development, late puberty
- Depression, irritability, difficulty concentrating, learning difficulties
- Reduced resistance to environmental pollutants and radiation
- Increased lipid peroxidation
- Poor sperm production, disordered ovulation, reduced fertility in both males and females
- Weakened immune response with increased infections

Laboratory Measurement of Status

Measure	Values	Comments
Serum zinc	Levels < 10.7 μmol/L indicate deficiency; levels 10.7–13.0 μmol/L indicate marginal status.	Levels are decreased in moderate to severe deficiency. Infection and/or stress may shift zinc from plasma to liver and decrease plasma levels without affecting body stores.
Zinc tolerance test	A two- to three-fold increase in plasma zinc indicates zinc deficiency.	After a baseline plasma zinc measurement, an oral load of 50 mg elemental zinc is given; 120 minutes later, plasma zinc is remeasured.

Good Dietary Sources

Food	Serving Size	mg
Calf liver	100 g	6–8
Oysters	100 g	>7
Lentils	100 g	5
Green peas	100 g	4
Whole wheat bread	100 g	2–4

Recommended Daily Intakes

Prevention of Deficiency			Therapeutic Dose Range
	UK RNI (1991)	USA RDA (1989)	Werbach (1990/99)
Men	9.5 mg	15 mg	20–150 mg
Women*	7 mg	12 mg	20–150 mg

* excluding pregnant or lactating women

Preferred Forms, Bioavailability, and Dosing

Organically-bound forms (zinc gluconate, orotate, protein hydrolysate, and chelated forms) generally have greater bioavailability than zinc sulfate.	Zinc supplements should usually be taken between meals. If gastrointestinal side effects occur, taking zinc with meals may reduce them.

Toxicity

Hathcock LOAEL (1997)
60 mg/day

Zinc is a nontoxic micronutrient at moderate supplementation levels (<100 mg/day). At doses of >150 mg, zinc may cause nausea and vomiting, and may interfere with copper absorption. At very high doses (>300 mg/day), zinc may impair immune function and may decrease HDL-cholesterol levels in the blood.

The Amino Acids

Arginine

Functions

- Release of hormones, including growth hormone, insulin, and adrenal norepinephrine
- Production of white blood cells
- Production of nitric oxide (nitric oxide regulates white blood cell function, vasodilation, and neurotransmission in the brain)
- Component of the urea cycle
- Synthesis of polyamines (spermine, spermidine) required for cell division and growth

Good Dietary Sources

Food	Serving Size	mg
Peanuts	100 g	3460
Soybeans	100 g	2200
Hazelnuts	100 g	2030
Shrimp	100 g	1740
Lamb, filet	100 g	1400

Recommended Daily Intakes

Recommended doses for arginine supplementation range from 1.5–6 g per day. Because the absorption of single high doses (>3 g) is poor, arginine supplements should be divided through the day. Because lysine competes with arginine for absorption and metabolism in the body, a diet low in lysine can enhance the effects of arginine supplementation.

Preferred Forms, Bioavailability, and Dosing

As a salt of L-arginine	Take in divided doses away from meals.

Toxicity

Doses of 1–6 g of arginine per day are generally well tolerated by healthy adults. High dose arginine supplementation may produce diarrhea, which is likely due to poor absorption of the arginine.

Branched-Chain Amino Acids: Leucine, Isoleucine, and Valine

Functions

- Energy source for muscle
- Decrease protein breakdown and encourage protein conservation and synthesis during times of increased physiological stress

Good Dietary Sources

Food	Serving Size	Valine (mg)	Leucine (mg)	Isoleucine (mg)
Peanuts	100 g	1450	2030	1230
Tuna	100 g	1420	2170	1210
Salmon	100 g	1390	1770	1160
Beef, filet	100 g	1150	1700	1090
Veal, filet	100 g	1120	1660	1110

Recommended Daily Intakes

In healthy people, the daily requirements for the branched-chain amino acids (BCAAs) to replace losses from normal protein metabolism and turnover are:

Valine	10 mg/kg body weight
Isoleucine	10 mg/kg body weight
Leucine	14 mg/kg body weight

During physiological stress, requirements for BCAAs are sharply increased (up to 5–10 g/day). Supplemental BCAAs are usually given in the range of 1–10 g/day, and are best absorbed when taken on an empty stomach. Intravenous doses range from 0.5–1.5 mg/kg/day.

Preferred Forms, Bioavailability, and Dosing

As a salt of L-valine, L-leucine, or L-isoleucine	Take in divided doses away from meals.

Toxicity

High doses of the BCAAs may decrease transport into the brain of tryptophan, the precursor to serotonin. People with conditions that may be aggravated if serotonin levels are lowered (insomnia, depression, migraine) should be cautious with high doses of the BCAAs.

Carnitine

Carnitine can be obtained from the diet or synthesized in cells by joining methionine and lysine, a process that requires vitamins C, B6, and niacin (vitamin B3). During periods of increased demand or increased loss, body synthesis of carnitine may be inadequate to supply needs, and carnitine from the diet (or supplements) becomes essential.

Functions

- Oxidation of fatty acids for energy
- Liver detoxification and excretion of chemicals and drugs

Increased Risk of Deficiency

- High fat diets
- Increased physiological stress: strenuous exercise, illness and infection, trauma
- Inadequate amounts of the precursors for carnitine synthesis—lysine and methionine, and vitamins C, B6, and niacin (vitamin B3)
- Pregnancy and lactation

Good Dietary Sources

Food	Serving Size	mg
Beef, filet	100 g	3680
Ground beef	100 g	3615
Pork chop	100 g	1075
Cod	100 g	210
Chicken, breast	100 g	150

The average adult diet that includes meat, milk, and eggs provides about 100–300 mg of carnitine per day. Animal foods are rich in carnitine, but plant foods are not: vegetables, fruits, and cereals have negligible amounts. Because dietary carnitine is practically absent from strict vegetarian diets, vegetarians are at increased risk of deficiency.

Recommended Daily Intakes

Supplemental carnitine is usually administered in oral doses ranging from 1–3.5 g/day.

Preferred Forms, Bioavailability, and Dosing

As a salt of L-carnitine (Only pure L-carnitine should be used as a supplement; D-carnitine can interfere with the action of L-carnitine in the body and produce signs of deficiency.)	Take in divided doses away from meals.

Toxicity

L-carnitine in doses of up to 4 g/day has no side effects other than occasional and temporary diarrhea. There have been reports that DL-carnitine (containing the potentially toxic D-isomer) can produce muscle weakness. Only L-carnitine should be used as a supplement.

Cysteine and Glutathione

Cysteine can function independently as an antioxidant or be combined with glutamic acid and glycine in the liver to form glutathione. The dietary supply of cysteine is a primary determinant of glutathione synthesis in the body. Supplements of cysteine can boost tissue levels of glutathione.

Functions

Cysteine:

- Antioxidant
- Detoxification of drugs and chemicals
- Cell membrane synthesis and repair
- Structural component of connective tissue

Glutathione:

- Antioxidant; recycles oxidized vitamins E and C
- Production of leukotrienes which modulate white blood cell activity and the inflammatory response

Good Dietary Sources

Because cysteine content of foods is difficult to measure, and methionine is the precursor of cysteine, food content of these two sulfur-containing amino acids is usually measured together. A table listing the best sources of these amino acids is shown on p. 72

Recommended Daily Intakes

In healthy adults, the daily requirement for cysteine and methionine needed to replace losses from normal protein metabolism is 13 mg/kg body weight. Recommended therapeutic doses for L-cysteine are in the range of 500–500 mg/day. If the primary aim of therapy is to increase glutathione levels, cysteine should be supplemented with glutamine and selenium.

Preferred Forms, Bioavailability, and Dosing

As a salt of L-cysteine (Because the absorption of glutathione supplements is unpredictable, cysteine supplements are the preferred method of increasing glutathione levels in the body. Supplements of L-cystine (formed by joining two cysteine molecules) should be avoided: they provide none of the antioxidant effects of cysteine and may increase the risk of kidney stones.)	Take in divided doses away from meals.

Toxicity

High doses of cysteine may be converted to cystine, and high levels of urinary cystine may increase risk the of kidney and bladder stones. Ample vitamin C intake (two to three times as much vitamin C as cysteine) helps prevent conversion of cysteine to cystine and reduces the chance of this side effect. Large doses of supplemental cysteine may interfere with the action of insulin and thereby worsen blood sugar control in diabetes; diabetics should consult their physician before taking large doses of cysteine. There are no published reports of toxicity from glutathione supplements.

Glutamine

Functions

- Precursor of gamma-aminobutyric acid (GABA), an inhibitory neurotransmitter
- Energy source for the cells lining the digestive tract and the white blood cells
- Conversion to glucose to maintain blood sugar levels
- Together with cysteine, precursor in the synthesis of glutathione

Good Dietary Sources

Food	Serving Size	mg
Ham	100 g	2860
Cheddar cheese	30 g	1600
Turkey, breast	100 g	1330
Chicken, breast	100 g	990
Milk	1 large glass	820

Recommended Daily Intakes

Oral glutamine supplements are normally taken in the range of 2–12 g/day.

Preferred Forms, Bioavailability, and Dosing

As a salt of L-glutamine	Take in divided doses away from meals.

Toxicity

Very high doses of glutamine may increase levels of glutamate in the brain, which can sometimes exacerbate mania or epilepsy. People who have these disorders should avoid large doses of glutamine.

Lysine

Functions

- Supports the immune system and has antiviral activity
- Precursor for carnitine synthesis

Good Dietary Sources

Food	Serving Size	mg
Tuna	100 g	2210
Pork loin	100 g	2120
Shrimp	100 g	2020
Beef, filet	100 g	2020
Soybeans	100 g	1900

Recommended Daily Intakes

In healthy adults, the daily requirement needed to replace losses from normal protein metabolism is 14 mg/kg body weight. Compared to adults, children have three times higher requirements for lysine per kilogram body weight; for example, recommendations for 10–12-year-old children are for 44 mg/kg body weight. Usual doses of lysine supplementation range from 0.5–4 g/day. Lysine and arginine share a common transport system for intestinal absorption and uptake into cells of the body and brain. Because arginine competes for uptake with lysine, a high ratio of lysine/arginine in the diet can enhance the effects of lysine supplementation.

Preferred Forms, Bioavailability, and Dosing

As a salt of L-lysine	Take in divided doses away from meals.

Toxicity

There are no reports of toxicity in healthy adults consuming lysine in the 1–4 g/day range.

Methionine

Functions

- The active form of methionine, S-adenosylmethionine (SAM), plays a central role in the synthesis of carnitine, choline, epinephrine, melatonin, and nucleic acids. It is particularly active in the brain. Low levels of SAM in the brain can produce lethargy and depression, and, when severe, psychiatric disorders.
- Dietary precursor to both cysteine and taurine.

Good Dietary Sources (Methionine and Cysteine*)

Food	Serving Size	mg
Salmon	100 g	700
Shrimp	100 g	670
Turkey, breast	100 g	630
Soybeans	100 g	580
Beef, filet	100 g	570

* Food content of the sulfur-containing amino acids methionine and cysteine is usually measured together

Recommended Daily Intakes

In healthy adults, the daily requirement for methionine and cysteine needed to replace losses from normal protein metabolism is 13 mg/kg body weight. Supplementation of methionine is normally in the 0.5–5 g range, and should be taken with vitamin B6.

Preferred Forms, Bioavailability, and Dosing

As a salt of L-methionine	Take in divided doses away from meals.

Toxicity

Large doses of methionine can be metabolized to homocysteine, a toxic metabolite. However, production of homocysteine is minimized by taking vitamin B6 along with methionine. High doses of methionine increase urinary excretion of calcium, and should be avoided by women with osteoporosis or at high risk of the disease. Very high doses in patients with schizophrenia may exacerbate hallucinations.

Phenylalanine and Tyrosine

The essential amino acid phenylalanine (PA) can be converted to tyrosine in the liver. However, during severe stress—infection, trauma, chronic illness, or liver disease—hepatic conversion of PA to tyrosine is impaired, and tyrosine becomes an essential amino acid.

Functions

- Precursor in the synthesis of the neurotransmitters dopamine, norepinephrine, and epinephrine
- Slows the breakdown of brain enkephalins (pain-reducing, opiate-like compounds)
- Precursor in production of the thyroid hormones

Good Dietary Sources (PA)

Food	Serving Size	mg
Soybeans	100 g	1970
Peanuts	100 g	1540
Almonds	100 g	1140
Tuna	100 g	1050
Beef, filet	100 g	930

Recommended Daily Intakes

In healthy people, the daily requirement for PA and tyrosine needed to replace losses from normal protein metabolism is 14 mg/kg body weight. Supplemental PA is usually given in daily doses ranging from 200 mg–8 g. Supplemental tyrosine is given in doses of from 200 mg–

6 g. PA and tyrosine should generally not be given concurrently, as the risk of side effects may be increased. Conversion of these amino acids to neurotransmitters in the brain can be enhanced if they are given together with vitamin B6.

Preferred Forms, Bioavailability, and Dosing

As a salt of L-tyrosine or L-phenylalanine (Supplemental amino acids should nearly always be given as the L-form [the naturally-occurring isomer], but because the D-form of PA has unique actions on pain pathways in the brain, supplements of PA taken for this purpose should be in the form of D,L-PA. For treatment of conditions other than chronic pain, the L-PA form is preferable and effective.)	Take in divided doses away from meals.

Toxicity

Supplemental PA and tyrosine may cause headaches, anxiety, or high blood pressure in rare cases. They should not be used by pregnant or lactating women, or phenylketonurics. High levels of PA and tyrosine in the blood of people with severe liver disease may contribute to mental impairment (encephalopathy) and coma. PA and tyrosine supplements should be avoided by people receiving monoamine oxidase (MAO) inhibitor-type antidepressants, as PA and tyrosine can dangerously raise blood pressure when taken with these drugs. PA and tyrosine supplements should also be avoided by schizophrenics, particularly those with high brain dopamine levels, as supplements may further increase brain dopamine and aggravate symptoms.

Taurine

Functions

- Growth and development of the brain and eye
- Component of several proteins and neurotransmitters important in the regulation of nervous function
- Stabilizer of excitable membranes in the heart, nerves, and platelets
- Antioxidant
- Binds to and detoxifies chemicals, drugs, and other xenobiotics in the liver
- Essential for proper bile acid function and fat absorption

Good Dietary Sources

Food	Serving Size	mg
Clams, fresh	100 g	240
Tuna	100 g	70
Oysters	100 g	70
Pork loin	100 g	50
Lamb, filet	100 g	47

Because taurine is virtually absent from plant foods, vegetarians have very low intakes.

Recommended Daily Intakes

Normal endogenous synthesis of taurine is estimated to be about 50–125 mg/day. Supplemental taurine is usually given in the range of 0.5–4.0 g/day.

Preferred Forms, Bioavailability, and Dosing

As a salt of taurine	Take in divided doses away from meals.

Toxicity

Taurine supplements can occasionally cause stomach irritation and may cause drowsiness in children. Otherwise, there are no reports of toxicity.

Tryptophan

Functions

- Precursor of serotonin (neurotransmitter which may induce mild drowsiness, improve mood, and reduce appetite);
- Niacin (vitamin B3) can be formed from tryptophan when dietary intake of preformed niacin is low.

Good Dietary Sources

Food	Serving Size	mg
Cashew nuts	100 g	450
Veal, filet	100 g	350
Sunflower seeds	100 g	310
Tuna	100 g	300
Chicken, breast	100 g	270

Recommended Daily Intakes

In healthy adults, the daily requirement needed to replace losses from normal protein metabolism is 3.5 mg/kg body weight. Tryptophan is the least abundant essential amino acid in the food supply. Because dietary levels of tryptophan are low relative to other amino acids, supplementation with even 500 mg is a substantial dietary increase. Supplemental tryptophan is generally given in the 500 mg–3 g range. Tryptophan's ability to raise brain serotonin levels is enhanced by concurrent ingestion of a small amount of carbohydrate (the insulin released in response to the carbohydrate will move valine, leucine, and isoleucine out of the blood into muscle, so competition for brain tryptophan uptake will be reduced). Ample vitamin B6 and riboflavin (vitamin B2) is required for production of serotonin (or niacin) from tryptophan.

Preferred Forms, Bioavailability, and Dosing

As a salt of L-tryptophan	Take in divided doses away from meals.

Toxicity

Use of certain tryptophan supplements in the 1980s was associated with the eosinophilia-myalgia syndrome (EMS). This syndrome was characterized by abnormal accumulation of eosinophils in connective tissue, muscle and joint pains, and excessive deposition of collagen in skin. In severe cases, EMS resulted in impaired brain function, disability, and death. The tryptophan that caused EMS all originated from a single manufacturer. It appears that the manufacturing process produced altered compounds, including abnormal forms of altered tryptophan that may have been responsible for causing the syndrome. It is very unlikely that pure tryptophan can cause EMS, but tryptophan supplements remain unavailable in many countries.

The Fats

Choline and Lecithin

The term lecithin is used in two ways. In chemistry, lecithin is another name for phosphatidylcholine, which contains about 13% choline by weight. In nutrition, lecithin is commonly used as the term for a substance typically derived from soybeans that contains a mixture of phosphatidylcholine (usually about 25%), myo-inositol, and other phospholipids.

Functions

- Formation of cell membranes and myelin
- Synthesis of acetylcholine in the peripheral and central nervous systems
- Liver metabolism of triglycerides and fats

Increased Risk of Deficiency

- High consumption of alcohol
- Low dietary intake of folate or conditions of impaired folate status, including chronic use of antibiotics, aspirin, oral contraceptive pills, chronic illnesses (liver disease, alcoholism, anemia), vitamin B12 deficiency
- Fat malabsorption
- HIV disease, AIDS

Signs and Symptoms of Deficiency

- Fat accumulation in the liver leading to liver damage
- Impaired kidney function
- Infertility
- Decreased hematopoesis
- Hypertension
- Abnormal growth
- Impairments in learning and memory
- Impairment in carnitine metabolism
- May increase risk of liver cancer

Good Dietary Sources

Food	Serving Size	mg
Calf liver	100 g	520
Eggs	1, medium size	270
Peanuts	100 g	95
Beef, filet	100 g	66
Cauliflower	100 g	42

Recommended Daily Intakes

	USA DRI (1998)
Men	550 mg
Women*	425 mg

* except pregnant and lactating women

Supplemental choline is usually taken in the 0.5–1.5 g/day range, while supplementation with lecithin is typically in the 2–10 g/day range.

Preferred Forms, Bioavailability, and Dosing

Lecithin (contains 20–25 % phosphatidylcholine by weight)	Take with meals

Toxicity

USA UI (1998)
3500 mg/day

Very high doses of choline (>20 g/day for several weeks) may produce nausea, vomiting, dizziness, and a fishy body odor. Lower doses (1–10 g) of choline have not been reported to cause toxicity. High doses of choline may produce depression in rare cases.

Essential Fatty Acids: Omega-3 and Omega-6 Fatty Acids

The two essential polyunsaturated fatty acids (PUFAs) are linoleic acid and linolenic acid. Linoleic acid is a member of the ω (omega)–6 fatty acid family, while linolenic acid is part of the ω (omega)–3 fatty acid group.

Functions

- *Components of cell membranes:*
  Incorporation increases membrane fluidity, cell responsiveness, and function
- *Formation of eicosanoids:*
  n-6 eicosanoids. Dietary linoleic acid can be converted into gamma-linolenic acid (GLA) in cells; GLA can then be further metabolized to form the n-6 group of eicosanoids. One of the most important is the prostaglandin PGE1, which reduces inflammation
  n-3 eicosanoids. Linolenic acid can be desaturated and elongated by cells to form the omega-3 fatty acids, eicosapentaenoic acid (EPA) and docosahexanoic acid (DHA). These fats are then metabolized into eicosanoids that reduce inflammation, dilate blood vessels, and decrease aggregation of platelets

Increased Risk of Deficiency

- Diets rich in meat and milk products but low in plant oils, fish, and seafood
- Deficiencies of zinc, magnesium, and vitamin B6 impair cell production of GLA, EPA, and DHA
- Older age groups
- Fat malabsorption: liver or biliary disease, Crohn disease, chronic pancreatitis, cystic fibrosis
- Major physiological stress due to injury, chronic illness, or surgery
- Rapid growth: pregnancy, childhood, and adolescence

Signs and Symptoms of Deficiency

- Dry, scaly skin, hair loss, and poor wound healing
- Impaired vision
- In childhood, reduced growth and impaired brain and eye development

- Infertility
- Reduced liver and kidney function, hematuria
- Increased fragility of red blood cells
- Reduced immune function, increased vulnerability to infections
- May increase risk of high blood pressure
- May increase risk of atherosclerosis and venous thrombosis
- May increase risk of inflammatory disorders, such as rheumatoid arthritis

Laboratory Measurement of Status

Measure	Values	Comments
PUFAs of the n-6 series		
Triene (20:3 n-9) to tetraene (20:4 n-6) ratio in blood	Ratio >0.4 indicates deficiency.	A sensitive indicator of deficiency.
PUFAs of the n-3 series		
Measurement of n-3 fatty acids in red blood cell membranes	Low levels (reference ranges vary between laboratories) indicate deficiency.	A sensitive indicator of deficiency.

Good Dietary Sources

Linoleic Acid	GLA
Vegetable oils (corn, safflower, soybean, sesame, sunflower)	Evening primrose oil (EPO) (contains about 10% GLA and 70% linolenic acid), borage oil, blackcurrant oil

Linolenic Acid	EPA and DHA
Soybeans, walnuts, wheat germ, linseeds, and their oils	Fish and shellfish, wild game. Fish oil capsules generally contain about 30% EPA and DHA.

Marine Sources of the Omega-3 Fatty Acids (mg/100 g of fish)

	EPA	DHA
Herring	2700	450
Tuna	1070	2280
Salmon	700	2140
Mackerel	690	1300
Halibut	190	500
Brook trout	150	335
Lobster	280	130
Shrimp	215	150

Recommended Daily Intakes

Prevention of Deficiency		Therapeutic Dose Range
	UK (1991)	Various authors
omega-3 fatty acids	0.2% of total calories	1–10 g of EPA and DHA* (3–30 g of fish oil)
omega-6 fatty acids	1% of total calories	100–600 mg GLA (1–6 g of EPO)

* recommended intake of EPA and DHA varies according to the indication:

1. As a daily supplement in healthy people who rarely eat fish, to maintain a balanced intake of fats, fish oil supplements are usually taken in the 0.5–1.0 g/day range.
2. For people with chronic ailments that may benefit from increasing omega-3 intake (see below), supplements are usually in the range of 2–4 g/day.
3. For high-dose, acute therapy for serious illness or recovery from injury or major surgery, supplements are given in the range of 3–30 g/day.

Preferred Forms, Bioavailability, and Dosing

Omega-3 fatty acids	As fish oil capsules containing vitamin E as an antioxidant.	Take with meals, preferably with the dose divided throughout the day.
Omega-6 fatty acids	Although borage oil has a higher concentration of GLA, EPO is generally preferable in that it contains an optimal range of fatty acids. Capsules of EPO should contain vitamin E as an antioxidant.	Take with meals, preferably with the dose divided throughout the day.

Toxicity

High doses of EFAs without additional vitamin E intake can deplete body stores of vitamin E. In some diabetics, high doses of omega-3 fatty acids can reduce insulin action and elevate blood sugar. In individuals with rare inherited bleeding disorders or those taking anticoagulant drugs, high-dose omega-3 supplementation may increase the risk of abnormal bleeding. People with epilepsy or mania should used GLA with caution. In rare cases, high dose supplementation may aggravate these disorders.

The Antioxidants

Antioxidants and Free Radicals

Sources of Free Radicals

- The respiratory chain in mitochondria
- The immune system
- Air pollution
- Cigarette smoke
- Radiation
- Excessive exposure to sunlight
- Industrial chemicals and solvents
- Medicines and drugs
- Herbicides and pesticides in foods
- Food additives: preservatives, colorings

Disorders Associated with Free Radical Damage

- Cancer
- Cardiovascular disease
- Adverse drug reactions
- Alcohol-induced liver damage
- Cataracts and macular degeneration
- Allergy and hypersensitivity
- Osteoarthritis and rheumatoid arthritis
- Inflammatory bowel disease (ulcerative colitis, Crohn disease)
- Neurological degeneration (multiple sclerosis, Parkinson disease)
- Ischemia/reperfusion injury after heart attack or stroke
- Trauma, surgery, or chronic infection
- Complications of diabetes mellitus
- Overuse injuries to muscles during intense exercise

Antioxidants

- Vitamin E
- Vitamin C
- Beta-carotene
- Glutathione
- Coenzyme Q10

- Cysteine
- Vitamin A

Antioxidant Enzymes and Their Vitamin and Trace Element Components

Antioxidant Enzymes	Trace Element
Glutathione peroxidases	Selenium
Catalase	Iron
Superoxide dismutases	Zinc, manganese, and copper
Glutathione reductase	Riboflavin (vitamin B2)

Laboratory Measurement of Status

Measure	Values
Plasma ascorbate	Levels < 23 μmol/L indicate deficiency.
Plasma beta-carotene	Normal levels are 0.3–0.6 μmol/L.
Serum total carotenoids	Levels < 50 μmol/L indicate deficiency.
Plasma vitamin E	Levels < 11.6 μmol/L indicate deficiency.
Plasma selenium	Normal range is 0.9–1.9 μmol/L.
Blood glutathione peroxidase	Activity < 30 E/g Hb indicates deficiency.
Erythrocyte Cu/Zn superoxide dismutase	Normal values are 0.47 ± 0.067 mg/g Hb.
Plasma coenzyme Q10	Normal levels are 0.4–1.0 μmol/L.

Recommended Daily Intakes

Vitamin C	250–500 mg
Vitamin E	100–200 mg
Beta-carotene	10–15 mg
L-cysteine	0.5–1 g
Coenzyme Q10	30–100 mg
Selenium	50–100 μg
Zinc	15 mg
Manganese	5–7.5 mg

Coenzyme Q10

Coenzyme Q10 can be obtained in small amounts from the diet or can be synthesized in cells. During periods of increased demand or increased loss, endogenous synthesis may be inadequate to supply needs and coenzyme Q10 from the diet becomes essential.

Functions

- Energy production in mitochondria
- Antioxidant

Laboratory Measurement of Status

Measure	Values
Plasma coenzyme Q10	Normal levels are 0.4–1.0 μmol/L.

Good Dietary Sources

Coenzyme Q10 is widely distributed in foods, but only in small amounts. Soybeans, walnuts, and almonds (and their oils), meats, certain fish (particularly abundant in mackerel and sardines), nuts, wheat germ, and some vegetables (e.g., green beans, spinach, cabbage, and garlic) are the best sources. Sardines are particularly rich in coenzyme Q10. However, it would be necessary to eat 1.6 kg of sardines to obtain 100 mg of coenzyme Q10. Therefore, in times of increased need, supplements of coenzyme Q10 may be the most efficient way to maintain body levels.

Recommended Daily Intakes

Usual supplementation with coenzyme Q10 is in the range of 30–120 mg/day. Supplementation with 60–100 mg in adults will double plasma levels of coenzyme Q10. Supplemental doses do not impair endogenous synthesis of coenzyme Q10.

Preferred Forms, Bioavailability, and Dosing

Coenzyme Q10	Take with meals

Toxicity

Even very large oral doses of coenzyme Q10 (600 mg/day) for prolonged periods do not appear to produce significant adverse side effects. Some people may experience mild nausea or gastrointestinal discomfort when taking coenzyme Q10.

II. Micronutrient Supplementation Through the Lifecycle

Women Considering Pregnancy

Women preparing for pregnancy need to build ample micronutrient reserves prior to conception. Combining a balanced diet with a high-quality multivitamin/mineral supplement is a good way to achieve this goal. Taking a multivitamin supplement containing 0.4–0.8 mg of folic acid during the months leading up to conception and the first months of pregnancy can sharply reduce the risk of birth defects, particularly neural tube defects.
Supplementation is particularly important for women who have been taking oral contraceptives. Birth control pills can interfere with metabolism of folate and vitamins B6 and B12. A woman planning for a pregnancy should stop taking oral contraceptives at least 3–6 months before planned conception, and substitute another form of birth control. During this period, a multivitamin/mineral supplement (containing ample amounts of the B vitamins and at least 0.4 mg of folate) should be taken to replenish body stores in preparation for pregnancy.

Vitamins	Recommended Daily Dose	Minerals	Recommended Daily Dose
Vitamin A	800 µg	Calcium	600–800 mg
Vitamin D	10–15 µg	Magnesium	300–400 mg
Vitamin E	15–20 mg	Iron	10–20 mg
Vitamin K	75–150 µg	Zinc	15 mg
Thiamin (vitamin B1)	1.5–2 mg	Iodine	200 µg
Riboflavin (vitamin B2)	1.6–2.2 mg	Selenium	100–150 µg
Niacin (vitamin B3)	20 mg	Copper	2 mg
Vitamin B6 Pantothenic acid	2.5–5 mg 5–10 mg	Manganese Fluoride	2–5 mg 1–3 mg*
Biotin	75–150 µg	Chromium	100–200 µg
Folic acid	0.8 mg	Molybdenum	100–250 µg
Vitamin B12	3–5 µg		
Vitamin C	100 mg		

* Not necessary if the local water or salt supply is fluoridated.

References

Block G et al. Vitamin and mineral status of women of childbearing potential. *Ann N Y Acad Med.* 1993; 678:245.

Centers for Disease Control and Prevention. Recommendations for the use of folic acid to reduce the number of cases of spina bifida and other neural tube defects. *MMWR.* 1992; 41:14.

Keen CL et al. Should vitamin-mineral supplements be recommended for all women of childbearing potential? *Am J Clin Nutr.* 1994; 59:532.

Pregnancy and Lactation

While the energy requirement during pregnancy and lactation increases by only 15–20%, needs for many micronutrients increase by 50–100%. The diets of most pregnant women do not cover these increased needs; intake of vitamins B6, D, E, and folate, and the minerals iron, calcium, zinc, and magnesium is often inadequate. Over two thirds of pregnant women show signs of one or more nutrient deficiencies. A balanced multivitamin/mineral reduces the risk of birth defects such as neural tube defects and cleft palate. It also can help prevent maternal anemia, diabetes, and hypertension. A complete multivitamin/mineral supplement is a sensible part of any healthy pregnancy.
The key to nutritional supplementation during pregnancy is balance. Many pregnant women receive a supplement containing high doses of iron and folic acid, but insufficient zinc. Both folic acid and iron reduce the absorption of zinc—and a deficiency of zinc can increase the risk of complications during pregnancy. Mineral intake should be balanced, with the optimal ratios of zinc to copper, as well as calcium to phosphorus and magnesium.
Because maternal needs for most micronutrients are even higher during lactation than in pregnancy, it is important to continue taking a multivitamin/mineral supplement after delivery. This will replenish nutrient stores depleted by the demands of pregnancy, and maintain nutrient stores to support milk production. Because breast milk is built from substrates obtained from the mother's bloodstream, the nutrition of the mother can have a substantial influence on the nutritional quality of her milk. Poor intake of vitamins or trace minerals by the mother can reduce the nutritional quality of her breast milk and produce deficiencies in her infant.

Recommended Daily Intake (Combined Intake from Food and Supplement Sources)

Vitamins		Minerals	
Vitamin A (preferably as beta-carotene)	800 µg	Calcium	1.5–2 g
Vitamin D	10–20 µg	Magnesium	400–600 mg

Vitamins		Minerals	
Vitamin E	20 mg	Iron	30 mg
Vitamin K	100 μg	Zinc	20–30 mg
Thiamin (vitamin B1)	2 mg	Copper	2–3 mg
Riboflavin (vitamin B2)	2 mg	Manganese	2–4 mg
Niacin (vitamin B3)	20 mg	Fluoride	2 mg
Vitamin B6	5 mg	Iodine	200 μg
Pantothenic acid	5–10 mg	Selenium	100–150 μg
Biotin	100–150 μg	Chromium	200 μg
Folic acid	0.8 mg	Molybdenum	200–250 μg
Vitamin B12	3 μg		
Vitamin C	100 mg		
Macronutrients			
Protein		70–90 g	
Essential fatty acids (linoleic and linolenic acids)		25–30 g	
Omega-3 fatty acids (eicosapentaenoic acid [EPA] and docosahexanoic acid [DHA])		4–6 g	
Fiber		25–30 g	

References

Belizan JM, Villar J, Gonzalez L, et al. Calcium supplementation to prevent hypertensive disorders of pregnancy. *N Engl J Med.* 1991; 325:1399.

Berger H, ed. *Vitamins and Minerals in Pregnancy and Lactation.* NNW Series. Vol.16. New York: Raven Press; 1988.

Cross NA et al. Calcium homeostasis and bone metabolism during pregnancy, lactation and postweaning: a longitudinal study. *Am J Clin Nutr.* 1995; 61:514.

Institute of Medicine. *Nutrition during Lactation.* Washington DC: National Academy Press; 1991.

Jovanovic-Peterson L, Peterson CM. Vitamin and mineral deficiencies which may predispose to glucose intolerance of pregnancy. *J Am Coll Nutr.* 1996; 15:14.

Keen CL et al, eds. Maternal Nutrition and Pregnancy Outcome. *Ann NY Acad Sci.* 1993; 678:1–367.

King JC, Sachet PP, Malpern GM, eds. Maternal Nutrition: New Developments and Implications. Am J Clin Nutr. 2000; 71 (S): 1217S–1375S

Lönnerdal B. Regulation of Mineral and Trace Elements in Human Milk: Exogenous end Endogenous Factors. Nutr Rev 2000; 58: 223–329

Swanson CA, King JC. Zinc and pregnancy outcome. *Am J Clin Nutr.* 1987; 46:763.

Viteri FE. The consequences of iron deficiency and anemia in pregnancy. In: Allen L, King J, Lonnerdal, eds. *Nutrient Regulation during Pregnancy, Lactation and Infant Growth.* New York: Plenum Press; 1994

Infancy (The First Year)

Vitamin D is particularly important for breastfed infants during the winter months in northern latitudes, when sunlight exposure is low. Iron intake from breast milk is inadequate to meet the needs of the rapidly growing infant after the fourth month, and supplemental iron is important until the infant is weaned onto iron-rich foods. The essential omega-3 fatty acids EPA and DHA are vital for the developing retina and nervous system of the newborn.

Nutrient	Recommended Daily Dose
Vitamin D	5 μg
Iron	10 mg
Omega-3 fatty acids with vitamin E	500 mg with 5 mg vitamin E
Fluoride	0.2 mg*

* only until the infant begins to receive fluoridated water or salt

References

Crawford MA. The role of essential fatty acids in neural development: implications for perinatal nutrition. *Am J Clin Nutr.* 1993; 57:703.
Fomon SJ. *Nutrition of Normal Infants.* St. Louis: Mosby Year Book Inc.; 1993.
Greer FR, Marshall S. Bone mineral content, serum vitamin D metabolite concentrations, and ultraviolet B light exposure in infants fed human milk with and without vitamin D2 supplements. *J Pediatr.* 1989; 114:204.
Sheard NF. Iron deficiency and infant development. *Nutr Rev.* 1994; 52:137.

Children and Adolescents

Most children's' and adolescents' diets are erratic and unpredictable, and persuading them to choose healthy foods can be difficult. Poor dietary intake combined with very high nutritional needs sharply increases the risk of micronutrient deficiencies. For many children, taking a well-balanced multivitamin/mineral supplement to ensure adequate micronutrient intake is important. However, a multivitamin/mineral supplement cannot replace healthy foods and good dietary habits. The diet should be high in fruits, vegetables, whole grains, and legumes. Dairy products, lean meats, poultry and fish are also important. Processed and refined foods should be avoided: most contain artificial additives, colorings, and flavorings, as well as high amounts of added sugar, salt, and hydrogenated fats. Healthy snacks, such as milk, yogurt, fruit, nuts, and wholegrain baked goods, should be available throughout the day.

1–3 Years of Age

Vitamins	Recommended Daily Dose	Minerals	Recommended Daily Dose
Vitamin A	400 µg	Calcium	500 mg
Vitamin D	10 µg	Magnesium	200 mg
Vitamin E	10 mg	Iron	10 mg
Vitamin C	50 mg	Zinc	10 mg
Thiamin (vitamin B1)	1 mg	Copper	1 mg
Riboflavin (vitamin B2)	1 mg	Selenium	20 µg
Niacin (vitamin B3)	10 mg	Iodine	50 µg
Vitamin B6	2 mg	Manganese	2 mg
Folic acid	50 µg	Fluoride*	1 mg
Vitamin B12	1 µg	Chromium	50 µg
Biotin	20 µg	Molybdenum	50 µg
Pantothenic acid	5 mg		

* only if the water or salt supply is not fluoridated

≥4 Years of Age and Adolescents

Vitamins	Recommended Daily Dose	Minerals	Recommended Daily Dose
Vitamin A	700 µg	Calcium	600 mg
Vitamin D	10 µg	Magnesium	300 mg
Vitamin E	20 mg	Iron	10–20 mg
Vitamin C	100 mg	Zinc	10–20 mg
Thiamin (vitamin B1)	2–5 mg	Copper	2–3 mg
Riboflavin (vitamin B2)	2–5 mg	Selenium	100 µg
Niacin (vitamin B3)	25–50 mg	Iodine	150 µg
Vitamin B6	10–15 mg	Manganese	2–5 mg
Folic acid	0.4 mg	Fluoride*	1–2 mg
Vitamin B12	2–5 µg	Chromium	100–200 µg
Biotin	50–100 µg	Molybdenum	150–250 µg
Pantothenic acid	5–10 mg		

* only if the water or salt supply is not fluoridated

References

Bruner AB et al. Randomised study of cognitive effects of iron supplementation in non-anemic iron-deficient adolescent girls. *Lancet* 1996; 348:992.

Castillo Duran C et al. Zinc supplementation increases growth velocity of male children and adolescents with short stature. *Acta Paediatr.* 1994; 83:833.

Caulfield LE et al. Nutritional supplementation during early childhood and bone mineralization during adolescence. *J Nutr.* 1995; 125:1104.

King J. Does poor zinc nutriture retard skeletal growth and mineralization in adolescents? *Am J Clin Nutr.* 1996; 64:375.

Middleman AB et al. Nutritional vitamin B12 deficiency and folate deficiency in an adolescent patient presenting with anemia, weight loss, and poor school performance. *J Adolesc Health.* 1996; 19:76.

Milner JA. Trace elements in the nutrition of children. *J Pediatr.* 1990; 117:147.

Oski FA. Iron deficiency in infancy and childhood. *N Engl J Med.* 1993; 329:190.

Teegarden D, Weaver CM. Calcium supplementation increases bone density in adolescent girls. *Nutr Rev.* 1994; 52:171.

Older Adulthood

Micronutrient supplementation is particularly beneficial in older age groups because many older people eat less and are less able to absorb micronutrients from foods. Moreover, in older adults, even mild deficiencies of micronutrients—such as vitamin B6, vitamin E, and zinc—can weaken the immune system. Deficiencies of vitamin B12 and thiamin (vitamin B1) are common among older adults and impair memory and concentration. Boosting intake of antioxidants—using micronutrient supplementation together with an optimal diet—can help protect against arthritis, heart disease, osteoporosis, and cataracts. Together with eating a well-balanced diet and keeping physically active, micronutrient supplementation can be a powerful tool to maintain function in the later years.

Compensating for Reduced Nutrient Absorption at Older Ages

	Recommended Daily Dose
Vitamin D	10–15 μg
Vitamin B6	20–25 mg
Vitamin B12	5 μg
Folic acid	0.4–0.8 mg
Calcium	1.5–2 g
Magnesium	500 mg
Zinc	10–20 mg

Antioxidant Protection Against the Chronic Degenerative Diseases

	Recommended Daily Dose
Vitamin C	1 g
Vitamin E	400 mg
Beta-carotene	15 mg
L-cysteine	1.5 g

	Recommended Daily Dose
Coenzyme Q10	100 mg
Selenium	200 μg
Zinc	20 mg
Manganese	10 mg

To Maintain Optimal Function of the Immune System

	Recommended Daily Dose
Vitamin B6	10–25 mg
Vitamin E	200–400 mg
Vitamin C	0.5–1 g
Zinc	10–15 mg
Selenium	50–100 μg
+ a balanced vitamin /mineral supplement	

Reducing the Risk of Osteoporosis

	Recommended Daily Dose
Vitamin D	10 μg
Calcium	1–2 g
Magnesium	400–600 mg
+ a balanced multimineral supplement	

References

Goodwin JS et al. Association between nutritional status and cognitive function in a healthy elderly population. *JAMA.* 1983; 249:2917.

Meunier P. Prevention of hip fractures by correcting calcium and vitamin D insufficiencies in elderly people. *Scand J Rheumatol.* 1996; Suppl. 103:75.

Monget AL et al. Effect of 6-month supplementation with different combinations of an association of antioxidant nutrients on biochemical parameters and markers of the antioxidant defence system in the elderly. The Geriatrie/Min.Vit.Aox Network. *Eur J Clin Nutr.* 1996; 50:443.

Russell RM, Suter PM. Vitamin requirements of elderly people: an update. *Am J Clin Nutr.* 1993; 58:4.

Tucker K. Micronutrient status and aging. *Nutr Rev.* 1995; 53:9.
Tucker KL et al. Folic acid fortification of the food supply. Potential benefits and risks for the elderly population. *JAMA.* 1996; 276:1879.
Wood RJ et al. Mineral requirements of elderly people. *Am J Clin Nutr.* 1995; 62:493.

III. Prevention and Therapy

Acquired Immunodeficiency Syndrome (AIDS)

Diet

In HIV infection, a critical determinant of disease progression is nutritional status. A combination of carefully-selected diet, prudent micronutrient supplementation, moderate exercise, and a supportive social environment can maintain optimal immune function and, along with effective drug therapy, help slow progression of the disease (see recommendations on p. 168 for infections). The diet should emphasize whole grains and fresh fruits and vegetables. Intake of refined carbohydrates, sugar, saturated fat, and alcohol should be sharply reduced. Foods rich in vitamins A, C, E, B6, and minerals zinc and selenium should be eaten regularly.

Micronutrients

Nutrient	Recommended Daily Dose	Comments
Vitamin A	3000–8000 μg as retinol or beta-carotene	Maintains the health of the skin and digestive tract epithelium, and can help reduce the risk of respiratory infection.
Vitamin C	500 mg–1 g	May help inhibit viral growth and maintain immune strength.
Vitamin B6	100–250 mg	Can enhance immune function and resistance to infection.
Vitamin E	200–400 mg	May reduce oxidant damage from infection and help maintain immune response to the virus.
Zinc	30–60 mg	Can enhance immune function and resistance to infection.
Selenium	200–300 μg	Deficiency sharply increases risk of progression and disease severity.
Arginine and glutamine	2–3 g arginine; 3–5 g glutamine	Arginine stimulates production of white blood cells; glutamine supports the immune system and increases white blood cell function.

References

Allard JP et al. Oxidative stress and plasma antioxidant micronutrients in humans with HIV infection. *Am J Clin Nutr.* 1998; 67:143.
Baum MK et al. High risk of HIV-related mortality is associated with selenium deficiency. *J Acquir Immune Def Syndr Hum Retrovirol.* 1997; 15:370.
Baum MK, Shor-Posner G. Micronutrient status in relationship to mortality in HIV-1 disease. *Nutr Rev.* 1998; 56:135.
Faluz J, Tsoukas C, Gold P. Zinc as a cofactor in human immunodeficiency virus-induced immuno-suppression. *JAMA.* 1988; 259:2850.
Gorbach SL et al. Interactions between nutrition and infection with HIV. *Nutr Rev.* 1993; 51:226.
Kalebic T et al. Suppression of human immunodeficiency virus expression in chronically infected monocytic cells by glutathione, glutathione ester, and N-acetylcysteine. *Proc Natl Acad Sci USA.* 1991; 88:986.
Ross AC, Stephenson CB. Vitamin A and retinoids in antiviral responses. *FASEB J.* 1996; 10:979.
Tang AM et al. Effects of micronutrient intake on survival in HIV-1 infection. *Am J Epidemiol.* 1996; 143:1244.

Acne

Diet

Excess consumption of saturated fats (fatty meat, whole milk, and chocolate) and hydrogenated fats (margarines and processed foods) can aggravate acne by increasing sebum production in the skin. Foods high in refined carbohydrates (particularly sucrose) and low in fiber can also stimulate sebum production. Food sensitivities (commonly to nuts and colas) can trigger acne in susceptible individuals. Acne can be caused by preparations containing iodine, such as kelp products and certain medicines.

To help reduce the frequency and severity of acne

Reduce or eliminate these foods:	Eat more of these foods:
Foods high in saturated fat: fatty meats, whole milk, cheese, butter, chocolate	Raw vegetables and wholegrain products
Foods high in hydrogenated fat: margarine, processed baked products (pastries, cookies)	Fresh fruit and fruit juice
Salty, fatty foods: potato chips, french fries	Fresh fish and other seafood
Nuts: particularly salted almonds and peanuts	
White flour and sugar, cola drinks	

Micronutrients

Nutrient	Recommended Daily Dose	Comments
Vitamin A	2000–10 000 μg	Can be effective in reducing severity and inflammation. High doses of vitamin A should only be taken under the advice of a physician.
Vitamin E and selenium	200–400 mg vitamin E; 200 μg selenium	Especially effective in treating pustules (whiteheads).

Nutrient	Recommended Daily Dose	Comments
Zinc	50–80 mg	Reduces inflammation and severity of acne.
Gamma-linolenic acid (GLA)	As 2–4 g evening primrose oil (EPO)	Reduces inflammation in the sebaceous glands. Take with 100 mg vitamin E.

References

Dreno B et al. Low doses of zinc gluconate for inflammatory acne. *Acta Derm Venereol Suppl Stockh.* 1989; 69:541.

Michaelsson G, Edqvist LE. Erythrocyte glutathione peroxidase activity in acne vulgaris, the effects of selenium and vitamin E treatment. *Acta Derm Venereol.* 1984; 64:9.

Pohit J et al. Zinc status of acne vulgaris patients. *J Appl Nutr.* 1985; 37:18.

Sherertz EF, Goldsmith LA. Nutritional Influences on the Skin. In: Goldsmith LA, ed. *Physiology, Biochemistry and Molecular Biology of the Skin.* Oxford: Oxford University Press; 1991.

Verm KC et al. Oral zinc sulfate therapy in acne vulgaris: A double-blind trial. *Acta Dermatovener.* 1980; 60:337–340

Ziboh VA. The significance of polyunsaturated fatty acids in cutaneous biology. *Lipids.* 1996; 31:249.

Alcohol Abuse

Diet

For most adults, occasional moderate alcohol drinking (one to two drinks per day) is not harmful, and may have health benefits. Moderate alcohol drinking can increase the HDL-cholesterol level in the blood, decrease the risk of blood clots, and may reduce the risk of a heart attack.
However, regular heavy drinking (more than three to four drinks per day) is a health hazard. (A 'drink' is defined as a 6 oz. glass of wine, a 12 oz. glass of beer, or 1–1.5 oz. of spirits.)

- Heavy drinking increases risk of high blood pressure, stroke, liver disease, immune weakness, and cancer.
- Heavy alcohol intake causes inflammation of the lining of the stomach and intestines, reducing the absorption of vitamins and minerals.
- Heavy drinking also damages the pancreas, which impairs production of digestive enzymes and further lowers nutrient absorption from foods.
- The liver is particularly vulnerable to alcohol—more than three drinks a day causes inflammation and accumulation of fat in the liver. This impairs liver function, reducing the ability to detoxify chemicals and drugs. Because the liver is important for blood sugar control, alcohol-induced liver damage can produce hypoglycemia, leading to fatigue, irritability, and difficulty concentrating.
- Alcohol increases urinary losses of many minerals, including zinc, calcium, and magnesium. Because of these effects, drinkers need to very carefully choose a diet rich in fresh fruits and vegetables, whole grains, lean meats, and low-fat milk products.
- Heavy alcohol intake during pregnancy, especially during the first 3 months, can cause birth defects and mental retardation in the infant. No one knows how much alcohol is safe during pregnancy, and many experts feel even one drink per day is harmful. The safest course for a pregnant woman is probably complete abstention during early pregnancy and only very rare intake in later pregnancy.

Micronutrients

To help prevent or reverse the damage done by alcohol

Nutrient	Recommended Daily Dose	Comment
Antioxidant formula	Containing vitamins A, C, E, zinc, and selenium	Alcohol can cause widespread cell damage and fat peroxidation in the liver. Supplements may help protect against oxidative damage. Vitamin C may help detoxify alcohol.
Vitamin B-complex	Complete formula containing at least 25 mg of vitamins B1, B2, B3, and B6, 0.4–0.8 mg of folic acid, and 25 μg of B12	B vitamins are poorly absorbed and their activation is impaired by alcohol. Most heavy drinkers are deficient in many B vitamins.
Carnitine	0.5–1.5 g	Reduces hepatic damage and development of fatty liver.
Niacinamide	1–1.5 g	Reduces damage to hepatic protein metabolism.
Magnesium	400 mg	Deficiency is very common in heavy drinkers, and can produce heart and neuromuscular problems.
Zinc	30–45 mg	The main enzymes that detoxify alcohol are dependent on zinc, thus zinc deficiency impairs ability to breakdown alcohol, increasing potential harm.

References

Odeleye OE, Watson RR. Alcohol-related nutritional derangements. In: Watson RR, Watzl B, eds. *Nutrition and Alcohol*. Boca Raton: CRC Press; 1992.

Chen MF et al. Effect of ascorbic acid on plasma alcohol clearance. *J Am Coll Nutr.* 1990; 9:185.

McClain CJ, Su L. Zinc deficiency in the alcoholic: A review. *Alcoholism*. 1983; 7:5.

Odeleye OE, Watson RR. Nicotinamide counteracts alcohol-induced impairment of hepatic protein metabolism in humans. *J Nutr.* 1997; 127:2199.

Ravel JM et al. Reversal of alcohol toxicity by glutamine. *J Biol Chem.* 1955; 214:497.

Sachan DS et al. Ameliorating effects of carnitine and its precursors on alcohol-induced fatty liver. *Am J Clin Nutr.* 1984; 39:738.

Salaspuro M. Nutrient intake and nutritional status in alcoholics. *Alcohol Alcoholism.* 1993; 28:85.

Segarnick DJ et al. Gamma-linolenic acid inhibits the development of the ethanol-induced fatty liver. *Prostaglandins Leukotrienes Med.* 1985; 17:277.

Shaw S, Lieber CS. Nutrition and diet in alcoholism. In: Shils ME, Young VR, eds. *Modern Nutrition in Health and Disease.* Philadelphia: Lea & Febiger; 1994.

Tanner AR et al. Depressed selenium and vitamin E levels in an alcoholic population: Possible relationship to hepatic injury through increased lipid peroxidation. *Dig Dis Sci.* 1986; 31:1307.

Allergic Rhinitis

Allergic rhinitis can be a manifestation of food sensitivity (see p. 146).

Micronutrients

Nutrient	Recommended Daily Dose	Comments
Vitamin C	250–750 mg	May increase breakdown of histamine produced as part of the allergic response, and thereby can help reduce allergic symptoms.
Niacin (vitamin B3)	100 mg	Reduces histamine production and release, and can help reduce allergic symptoms.
Calcium and magnesium	500 mg calcium and 250 mg magnesium (may be taken as dolomite tablets)	Calcium supplements can help reduce allergic responses. Magnesium deficiency may increase vulnerability to allergy.
Gamma-linolenic acid (GLA)	As 2–4 g evening primrose oil (EPO)	Reduces inflammation and congestion, rebalances the immune response.

References

Bucca C et al. Effect of vitamin C on histamine bronchial responsiveness of patients with allergic rhinitis. *Ann Allergy.* 1990; 65:311.

Horrobin DF, Morse PF. Evening primrose oil and atopic eczema. *Lancet.* 1995; 345:260.

Rolla G et al. Reduction of histamine-induced bronchoconstriction by magnesium in asthmatic subjects. *Allergy.* 1987; 42:286.

Anemia

Diet

The most common nutrient deficiencies that produce anemia are iron, folic acid, and vitamin B12. Less commonly, inadequate dietary supply of vitamins A and C, several other B vitamins, and copper produces anemia. Anemia due to deficiency of iron and folic acid is very common among growing children and pregnant women, because their diets do not supply adequate iron and folate to meet their increased needs. People with low iron stores should not drink coffee or black tea with their meals, as these beverages sharply reduce the absorption of iron from foods. Vitamin C strongly promotes absorption of iron, so a glass of orange juice or other vitamin C–rich food included with meals can be beneficial.

Micronutrients

Nutrient	Recommended Daily Dose	Comments
To prevent anemia and promote healthy development of red blood cells		
Vitamin B-complex	Should contain at least 5 mg vitamin B6, 0.4 mg folate, and 5 μg vitamin B12.	Lack of riboflavin (vitamin B2), thiamin (vitamin B1), folate, and vitamins B6 and B12 can all cause anemia. Particularly important during pregnancy and lactation, as well as during the childhood and teen years.
Multimineral supplement with iron	Containing balanced amounts of all essential minerals, including 5–10 mg iron.	Particularly important during pregnancy and lactation, as well as during the childhood and teen years. Vitamin C sharply increases absorption of iron when taken with an iron supplement.
To treat anemia due to a single nutrient deficiency		
Iron	100–150 mg elemental iron (in a bioavailable form, such as ferrous fumarate)	Iron supplements should be continued for 3–6 months after the hemoglobin level returns to normal, in order to refill iron stores.

Nutrient	Recommended Daily Dose	Comments
Folic acid	1–5 mg	Should be taken until hemoglobin returns to normal. Should be given along with a balanced vitamin B-complex containing at least 5 μg vitamin B12.
Vitamin B12	If due to vitamin B12 malabsorption: 1 mg via intramuscular injection/day for 7 days, then 1 mg intramuscularly twice per week for 2 months. If due to poor dietary intake (vegetarianism): 1 mg oral vitamin B12/day for 3–6 months.	After stores are replenished, vitamin B12 deficiency due to malabsorption usually requires lifelong monthly injections, or, in cases of mild malabsorption, 1 mg oral vitamin B12/day, to maintain status. For vegetarians, a daily supplement of 2–5 μg vitamin B12 will usually maintain reserves.

References

Ajayi OA, Nnaji UR. Effect of ascorbic acid supplementation on haematological response and ascorbic acid status of young female adults. *Ann Nutr Metab.* 1990; 34:32.

Beard JL et al. Iron metabolism: a comprehensive review. *Nutr Rev.* 1996; 54:295.

Hoffbrand AV. Megaloblastic anemia and miscellaneous deficiency anemias. In: Weatherall DJ, Ledingham JGG, Warrell DA, eds. *Oxford Textbook of Medicine.* Oxford: Oxford Medical Publications; 1996:3484–3500.

Hurrell RF. Bioavailability of iron. *Eur J Clin Nutr.* 1997; 51:4.

Lindenbaum J et al. Prevalence of cobalamin deficiency in the Framingham elderly population. *Am J Clin Nutr.* 1994; 60:2.

Middleman AB et al. Nutritional vitamin B12 deficiency and folate deficiency in an adolescent patient presenting with anemia, weight loss, and poor school performance. *J Adolesc Health.* 1996; 19:76.

Pruthi RK, Tefferi A. Pernicious anemia revisited. *Mayo Clin Proc.* 1994; 69:144.

Anxiety

Diet

In people susceptible to reactive hypoglycemia (see p. 166 ff.), consumption of refined carbohydrates or sugar may trigger increased anxiety and, in rare cases, panic attacks.

Micronutrients

Nutrient	Recommended Daily Dose	Comments
Tryptophan	1–3 g	Tryptophan can increase levels of serotonin, a brain chemical that has a calming effect. Should be taken together with 50 mg vitamin B6.
Niacinamide	500 mg–1 g	Has muscle relaxant and mild sedative effects and can reduce anxiousness.
Magnesium	400–600 mg	May decrease anxiety and nervous tension. Medications, illness, and stress can deplete magnesium stores and produce agitation and irritability.

References

Gorman JM et al. Hypoglycemia and panic attacks. *Am J Psychiatry.* 1984; 141:101.

Seelig MS. Consequences of magnesium deficiency on the enhancement of stress reactions; preventive and therapeutic implications (a review). *J Am Coll Nutr.* 1994; 13:429.

Young SN. Behavioral effects of dietary neurotransmitter precursors: basic and clinical aspects. *Neurosci Biobehav Rev.* 1996; 20:313.

Asthma

Diet

Asthma can be a symptom of food sensitivity, and can significantly improve if food sensitivities are diagnosed and offending foods eliminated (p. 146). Diets high in sodium may increase reactivity of the air passages to histamine, so asthmatics should minimize salt intake. Asthmatics should also avoid foods containing sulfite additives. Sulfites are added as preservatives to certain fresh vegetables, salads, potatoes, and wine, and they can trigger severe asthma.

Micronutrients

Nutrient	Recommend Daily Dose	Comments
Omega-3 fatty acids	2–4 g as fish oil capsules	Reduces inflammation and may decrease symptoms.
Magnesium	400 mg	Can reduce severity of attacks and improve lung function. Magnesium deficiency is commonly found among asthmatics.
Vitamin C	1–2 g	May increase breakdown of histamine produced as part of the asthmatic response, and may reduce frequency and severity of asthma. Can be particularly effective against asthma triggered by exercise.
Vitamin B6	50–100 mg	May reduce frequency and severity of asthmatic attacks.

References

Arm J et al. The effects of dietary supplementation with fish oil on asthmatic responses to antigen. *J Clin Allergy.* 1988; 81:183.

Bielory L, Gandhi R. Asthma and vitamin C. *Ann Allergy.* 1994; 73:89.

Blok WL. Modulation of inflammation and cytokine production by dietary (n-3) fatty acids. *J Nutr.* 1996; 126:1515.

Monem GF et al. Use of magnesium sulfate in asthma in childhood. *Pediatr Ann.* 1996; 25:139.

Reynolds RD, Natta CL. Depressed plasma pyridoxal phosphate concentrations in adult asthmatics. *Am J Clin Nutr.* 1985; 41:684.

Shimizu T et al. Theophylline attenuates circulating vitamin B6 levels in children with asthma. *Pharmacology.* 1994; 49:392.

Cancer

Diet

Dietary factors are estimated to play a role in about one half of all cases of cancer. Healthy dietary choices and prudent micronutrient supplementation may significantly reduce the risk of developing cancer. Maintaining a reasonable body weight is important: obesity increases the risk of cancer of the breast, colon, prostate, and uterus.
Different dietary factors have been identified as either cancer promoters or inhibitors.

Dietary substances that act as promoters:

- High intake of fat, especially saturated fat from meat products
- Processed meats (e.g., sausages, luncheon meats, smoked, pickled, or salt-cured meats)
- Burned or darkly browned foods, such as heavily roasted or barbecued meats
- Rancid (oxidized) fats, such as fat used repeatedly for deep-fat frying
- Nitrites and nitrates (food preservatives used to give processed meats a pink color)
- Old, moldy foods, particularly potatoes, peanuts, mushrooms, sprouts
- Pesticides and other agrochemicals
- Artificial food dyes (especially red-colored dyes)
- Regular heavy alcohol intake
- Heavily-chlorinated drinking water

Dietary substances that act as inhibitors:

- Fiber-rich foods (whole grains, bran, fruits, vegetables, legumes, seeds)
- Dark-green and yellow-orange vegetables
- The 'cruciferous' vegetables: broccoli, Brussels sprouts, cabbage, cauliflower
- Fresh beet, carrot, asparagus, and cabbage juices
- Onions and garlic
- Calcium-rich foods (e.g., low-fat dairy products)
- Fresh fruit and fruit juices

Micronutrients (to help reduce cancer risk)

Nutrient	Recommended Daily Dose	Comments
Selenium	200 μg	Supplementation reduces the risk of cancer. An essential component of antioxidant enzyme systems that can protect cells and DNA from oxidant damage. Deficiency increases the risk of developing cancer.
Vitamin A	1000 μg	Regulates healthy growth and development of the epithelium of the oropharynx, the digestive and respiratory tracts, and the skin. Supplementation may reduce the risk of cancer.
Vitamin C	250–500 mg	An antioxidant that helps protect cells and DNA from oxidant damage. Higher intakes reduce risk of cancer. Particularly effective in reducing risk of lung cancer and stomach cancer from processed meats containing nitrites.
Vitamin E	200 mg	An antioxidant that helps protect cell membranes and DNA from oxidant damage. May reduce risk of cancer.
Folic acid and vitamin B12	0.4 mg folic acid; 10–20 μg vitamin B12	Maintains healthy growth and development of the digestive and respiratory epithelium. May reduce the risk of cancer of the bronchi and lung, particularly in smokers.
Calcium and vitamin D	1 g calcium; 10 μg vitamin D	May reduce risk of developing colon cancer.

For treatment of cancer: Very high doses of vitamins A, C, E, and selenium are potentially beneficial as adjuvants in treatment of cancer. In addition, high-dose supplements of niacin (vitamin B3), vitamin E, and coenzyme Q10 can be particularly beneficial in reducing the toxicity of chemotherapy and radiation therapy. These treatments should be considered only in consultation with an oncologist.

References

Block G. Epidemiologic evidence regarding vitamin C and cancer. *Am J Clin Nutr.* 1991; 54:1310.

Bostick RM. Diet and nutrition in the etiology and primary prevention of colon cancer. In: Bendich A, Deckelbaum RJ, eds. *Preventive Nutrition.* Torowa, New Jersey: Humana; 1997:57–95.

Clark LC et al. Effects of selenium supplementation for cancer prevention in patients with carcinoma of the skin. *JAMA.* 1996; 276:1957.

DeCosse JJ et al. Effect of wheat fiber and vitamins C and E on rectal polyps in patients with familial adenomatous polyposis. *J Natl Can Inst.* 1989; 81:1290.

Dwyer JT. Diet and nutritional strategies for cancer risk reduction. Focus on the 21st century. *Cancer.* 193; 72:1024.

Fontham ETH. Prevention of upper gastrointestinal tract cancers. In: Bendich A, Deckelbaum RJ, eds. *Preventive Nutrition.* Torowa, New Jersey: Humana; 1997:33–55.

Garland CF et al. Can colon cancer incidence and death rates be reduced with calcium and vitamin D? *Am J Clin Nutr.* 1991; 54:193.

Heimburger DC et al. Improvement in bronchial squamous metaplasia in smokers treated with folate and vitamin B12. *JAMA.* 1988; 259:1525.

Stich HF et al. Remission of precancerous lesions in the oral cavity of tobacco chewers and maintenance of the protective effect of beta-carotene or vitamin A. *Am J Clin Nutr.* 1991; 53:298.

Trickler D, Shikler G. Prevention by vitamin E of experimental oral carcinogenesis. *J Natl Can Inst.* 1987; 78:165.

Willet WC, Hunter DJ. Vitamin A and cancers of the breast, large bowel and prostate: epidemiologic evidence. *Nutr Rev.* 1994; 52:53.

Carpal Tunnel Syndrome

Diet

Food sensitivities are an occasional cause of swelling in the wrists and can trigger carpal tunnel syndrome. An elimination diet (p. 146) can identify food sensitivities; avoiding the offending foods may provide significant relief.

Micronutrients

Nutrient	Recommended Daily Dose	Comments
Vitamin B6 and magnesium	100–200 mg vitamin B6, 400–600 mg magnesium	May reduce inflammation, swelling, and symptoms.
Thiamin (vitamin B1)	50–100 mg	May reduce inflammation and pain.
Vitamin E	400–800 mg	May reduce inflammation and symptoms.

References

Hanck A, Weiser H. Analgesic and anti-inflammatory properties of vitamins. *Int J Vitam Nutr Res.* 1985; 27:189.
Jacobson MD. Vitamin B6 therapy for carpal tunnel syndrome. *Hand Clin.* 1996; 12:253.
Skelton WP, Skelton NK. Thiamine deficiency neuropathy: it's still common today. *Postgrad Med.* 1989; 85:301.
Traber MG et al. Lack of tocopherol in peripheral nerves of vitamin E-deficient patients with peripheral neuropathy. *N Engl J Med.* 1987; 317:262.

Cataract

Diet

The risk of developing a cataract can be strongly influenced by diet and nutrient intake. Most cataracts are caused by oxidative damage from lifetime exposure of the lens to light and radiation entering the eye. The antioxidant vitamins A, C, and E are a major defense against oxidative damage, and eating foods rich in these nutrients each day can reduce the chances of developing cataract. Hyperlipidemia, diabetes, and obesity also increase the risk of developing cataract. All of these conditions are modifiable by dietary changes and nutritional supplementation.

Micronutrients

Nutrient	Recommended Daily Dose	Comments
Vitamin C	1–2 g	Vitamin C supplementation may slow or halt progression of early cataract.
Vitamin E	800 mg	To help prevent further clouding of the lens.
Riboflavin (vitamin B2)	50 mg (can be taken as part of a vitamin B-complex)	Riboflavin (vitamin B2) plays a crucial role in maintaining clarity of the lens, and may reduce clouding in mild cataract.
For prevention of cataract:		
Antioxidant formula	Generous amounts of vitamins A, C, and E, riboflavin (vitamin B2), and zinc (see p. 83 ff.)	Long-term supplementation helps prevent the development of cataract.

References

Bhat KS. Nutritional status of thiamine, riboflavin and pyridoxine in cataract patients. *Nutr Rep Int.* 1987; 36:685.

Jacques PF, Taylor A. Antioxidant status and risk for cataract. In: Bendich A, Deckelbaum RJ, eds. *Preventive Nutrition.* Totowa, New Jersey: Humana; 1997:267–284.

Jacques PF et al. Long-term vitamin C supplement use and prevalence of early age-related lens opacities. *Am J Clin Nutr* 1997; 66: 911–916.
Lyle BJ et al. Serum carotenoids and tocopherols and incidence of age-related nuclear cataract. *Am J Clin Nutr* 1999; 69: 272–277.

Cervical Dysplasia

Diet

A healthy diet can reduce the risk of developing cervical dysplasia (CD), and supplementation with micronutrients can help the dysplastic cells to revert to normal. A diet high in fat (particularly saturated fat from meat and whole milk products) increases the risk of CD, while a diet rich in fresh fruits and vegetables offers significant protection, probably due to its high content of vitamin C, carotenes, and fiber.

Micronutrients

Nutrient	Recommended Daily Dose	Comments
Vitamin A	3000 μg for women who have an abnormal Pap smear showing CD; 800 μg for prevention	May help reverse dysplasia. High doses of vitamin A should only be taken with the advice of a physician.
Folic acid	5 mg for women who have an abnormal Pap smear showing CD; 0.4 mg for prevention	May reverse dysplasia. Should be taken as part of a vitamin B-complex.
Vitamin B-complex	Balanced and complete, with at least 25 mg riboflavin (vitamin B2), vitamin B6, and pantothenic acid, and 25 μg vitamin B12	Deficiencies of riboflavin (vitamin B2), and vitamins B6 and B12 increase risk of CD. Supports health of lining cells of the cervix and vagina.
Antioxidant formula	Should contain ample beta-carotene, vitamin E, and vitamin C, as well as selenium (see p. 83 ff. for recommended daily intakes for antioxidants)	May help reverse cervical dysplasia. Low intake of antioxidants increases risk of developing CD.

References

Butterworth CE et al. Improvement in cervical dysplasia associated with folic acid therapy in users of oral contraceptives. *Am J Clin Nutr.* 1982; 35:73.
Childers JM et al. Chemoprevention of cervical cancer with folic acid. *Cancer Epidemiol Biomarkers Prev.* 1995; 4:155.
Giuliano AR, Gapstur S. Can cervical dysplasia and cancer be prevented with nutrients? *Nutr Rev.* 1998; 56:9.
Palan PR et al. Plasma levels of antioxidant beta-carotene and alpha-tocopherol in uterine cervix dysplasias and cancer. *Nutr Cancer.* 1991; 15:13.
Romney SL et al. Plasma vitamin C and uterine cervical dysplasia. *Am J Obstet Gynecol.* 1985; 151:976.
Shimizu H et al. Decreased serum retinol levels in women with cervical dysplasia. *Br J Cancer.* 1996; 73:1600.
Whitehead N et al. Megaloblastic changes in the cervical epithelium associated with oral contraceptive therapy and reversal with folic acid. *JAMA.* 1973; 226:1421.

Cigarette Smoking

Diet

Smoking can increase blood LDL-cholesterol levels, as well as increase oxidant damage to cholesterol, and increase the risk of heart attack and stroke. Smokers need to minimize intake of saturated fat and hydrogenated fat to help control their blood cholesterol level. Metabolism and breakdown of vitamin C in smokers is sharply increased (a pack of cigarettes uses up about 300 mg of the body's stores). Smokers need more than double the amount of vitamin C than nonsmokers to maintain body levels of the vitamin. Chronic vitamin C deficiency in smokers promotes bleeding gums, premature wrinkling of skin, and may increase the susceptibility of LDL-cholesterol to oxidation. Smoking also impairs metabolism of vitamin A, folate, and vitamin B12. Poor folate and vitamin B12 status in smokers increases their already high risk of developing cancer of the lung. Smoking interferes with conversion of vitamin B6 to its active form. Smoking also increases losses of calcium from the skeleton and may increase the risk of osteoporosis.

Micronutrients

To reduce the damage from cigarette smoke

Nutrient	Recommended Daily Dose	Comments
Antioxidant formula	Containing ample amounts of vitamins A, C, E (at least 100 mg), zinc, and selenium.	Cigarette smoke is a powerful oxidant causing widespread cell damage and may accelerate atherosclerosis and other degenerative changes in the skin, lungs, and other organs. Vitamin E requirements are higher in smokers; supplementation may help reduce oxidative damage.
Vitamin B-complex	Complete formula containing 0.4–0.8 mg folic acid and 25–50 μg B12	Supplements of folate and vitamin B12 can reduce the severity of the precancerous changes in the lungs of regular smokers.
Vitamin C	500 mg	Smoking breaks down body stores of vitamin C rapidly. May help reduce oxidative damage and loss of respiratory function.

References

Anderson R et al. Regulation by the antioxidants ascorbate, cysteine and dapsone of the increased extracellular and intracellular generation of reactive oxidants by activated phagocytes from cigarette smokers. *Am Rev Resp Dis.* 1987; 135:1027.

Brown KM et al. Erythrocyte membrane fatty acid composition of smokers and non-smokers: effects of vitamin E supplementation. *Eur J Clin Nutr.* 1998; 52:145.

Heimburger DC et al Improvement in bronchial squamous metaplasia in smokers treated with folate and B12. *JAMA.* 1988; 259:1525.

Marangon K et al. Diet, antioxidant status and smoking habits in French men. *Am J Clin Nutr.* 1998: 67:231.

Ness AR et al. Vitamin C status and respiratory function. *Eur J Clin Nutr.* 1996: 50:573.

Paiva SAR et al. Assessment of vitamin A status in chronic obstructive pulmonary disease patients and healthy smokers. *Am J Clin Nutr.* 1996; 64:928.

Preston AM. Cigarette smoking; nutritional implications. *Prog Food Nutr Sci.* 1991; 15:183.

Schectman G. Estimating ascorbic acid requirements for cigarette smokers. *Ann NY Acad Sci.* 1993; 686:335.

Stryker WS. The relation of diet, cigarette smoking and alcohol consumption to plasma beta-carotene and alpha-tocopherol levels. *Am J Epidemiol.* 1988; 127:283.

Van Antwerpen VL et al. Vitamin E, pulmonary functions and phagocyte-mediated oxidative stress in smokers and nonsmokers. *Free Rad Biol Med.* 1995; 18:935.

Vermaak WJH et al. Vitamin B6 status and cigarette smoking. *Am J Clin Nutr.* 1990; 51:1058.

Common Cold and Influenza

Diet

See the recommendations for infections on p. 168. Drinking plenty of hot fluids usually helps relieve congestion and clears secretions from the nose and throat.

Micronutrients

Nutrient	Recommended Daily Dose	Comments
Zinc	15–30 mg to help prevent colds. At the first sign of a cold developing, 60–90 mg as 15 mg doses divided between four to six doses throughout the day. Particularly effective in the form of tablets or lozenges that should be allowed to dissolve slowly in the mouth before swallowing.	Can effectively shorten the duration of a cold and reduce the severity of symptoms.
Vitamin C	250–500 mg to help protect against colds. 1 g to help treat a cold.	Can help reduce the severity and shorten the duration of a cold.

References

Hemilia H. Vitamin C intake and susceptibility to the common cold. *Br J Nutr.* 1997; 77:59.

Mossad SB et al. Zinc gluconate lozenges for treating the common cold. *Ann Intern Med.* 1996; 125:81.

Conjunctivitis

Diet

Consume foods such as carrots, canteloupe, liver, oranges, strawberries, and broccoli that are rich sources of vitamins A and C.

Micronutrients

Nutrient	Recommended Daily Dose	Comments
Vitamin A	5000 μg	Supports healing of the conjunctiva.
Vitamin C	500 mg–1 g	Enhances immune response to infection. Take until redness clears.
Zinc	60 mg	Supports healing and enhances the immune response. Take until redness clears.

References

Grimble RF. Effect of antioxidative vitamins on immune function with clinical applications. *Int J Vit Nutr Res* 1997; 67:312–320.

Shankar AH, Prasad AS. Zinc and immune function: the biological basis of altered resistance to infection. *Am J Clin Nutr* 1998; 68(S): 447S–63S.

Constipation and Diverticulitis

Diet

Constipation and diverticulitis are so-called „diseases of civilization," occurring in near epidemic proportions in the industrialized countries, where one fifth of the adult population suffers from chronic constipation, and diverticulosis occurs in about one third of people over 65 years old. The primary cause of both constipation and diverticulosis is a highly refined and processed diet that is low in dietary fiber. Dietary fiber passes into the colon intact and absorbs water—increasing the bulk of the stool and softening it. This stimulates peristalsis in the colon, pushing the stool forward more rapidly. Dietary fiber is found in large amounts in whole grains, corn, vegetables, fruits (dried prunes, apples, raisins, and figs), seeds, and legumes. Increasing intake of these foods will soften the stool and often eliminate constipation. Supplements of fiber, such as corn or wheat bran and psyllium seed preparations, can also be beneficial. However, because large amounts of fiber can produce gas and abdominal discomfort, fiber intake should be increased gradually as tolerated over a period of several weeks. Ample fluid intake (8–10 large glasses per day) should accompany increases in dietary fiber. In some people, high-dose calcium supplements (> 2 g/day) may worsen constipation.

Micronutrients

Nutrient	Recommended Daily Dose	Comments
Vitamin C	250 mg–2 g	Pulls water into the colon and softens the stool. Start with 250 mg and increase gradually until constipation improves. Take as single dose on arising in the morning.
Fiber	5–10 g	As psyllium supplements and/or from fresh/dried fruit. Take with ample water. Start with 1–2 g and increase as tolerated.
Vitamin B-complex	High potency containing 0.4–0.8 mg folic acid	Folic acid deficiency can aggravate constipation.

References

Cranston D et al. Dietary fibre and gastrointestinal disease. *Br J Surg.* 1988; 75:508.
Yang P, Banwell JG. Dietary fiber: Its role in the pathogenesis and treatment of constipation. *Practical Gastroenterology.* 1986; 6:28.

Coronary Heart Disease and Artherosclerosis

Diet

- *Dietary fat*
  Eating saturated fat raises levels of LDL-cholesterol, lowers HDL-cholesterol, and increases the tendency for platelet aggregation. Substituting polyunsaturated fats from nut and seed oils or monounsaturated fats from olive, peanut, and canola oil helps lower levels of LDL-cholesterol.
- *Hydrogenated fat*
  Hydrogenated oils are found in many processed baked goods and snacks, such as margarines and potato chips. They are as atherogenic as saturated fat, and intake should be minimized.
- *Dietary cholesterol*
  Blood cholesterol levels are much more influenced by the amount of saturated fat in the diet than by intake of dietary cholesterol. For people with normal values of blood cholesterol, dietary cholesterol has little effect on blood cholesterol levels. However, many people who are hypercholesterolemic can benefit from eating less cholesterol.
- *Fiber*
  Vegetables, fruits, beans, and whole grains are high in fiber. Fiber lowers blood cholesterol, and the soluble fiber found in fruits, oats, and vegetables is particularly beneficial.
- *Fish*
  Fish are rich in omega-3 fatty acids, which can lower blood cholesterol and triglycerides, lower blood pressure, and reduce platelet aggregation. Fish are also rich in protein and B vitamins, and low in saturated fat. Eating fish two to three times per week as part of a healthy diet can cut in half the risk of developing heart disease.
- *Dietary antioxidants*
  Antioxidants, both within lipoproteins (such as vitamin E) and circulating in the blood (beta-carotene and vitamin C) help protect against oxidation of blood lipids. Regular, daily intake of citrus fruits and green and yellow vegetables supplies these vitamins, as well as other important antioxidant food compounds.
- *B vitamins*
  Homocysteine, an amino acid that is a toxic byproduct of cell metabolism, can damage the lining of blood vessels and promote atheros-

clerosis. An elevated blood homocysteine level increases the risk of heart attack and stroke by two to five times. Vitamins B6, B12, and folate are essential for metabolism and clearance of homocysteine.

Micronutrients

Nutrient	Recommended Daily Dose	Comments
To reduce elevated blood homocysteine		
Folic acid and vitamin B12	0.5–1 mg folic acid; 10–20 μg vitamin B12	Reduces blood homocysteine levels.
Vitamin B6	50 mg	Reduces blood homocysteine levels; lowers risk of platelet aggregation.
To reduce elevated blood cholesterol		
Niacin (vitamin B3) (in form of nicotinic acid)	Begin with 100 mg and gradually increase over several weeks to 1–3 g. Take with meals	Lowers LDL-cholesterol and raises HDLs, thereby reducing the risk of heart attack. Side effects (flushing) can be minimized by raising the dose gradually and taking the niacin (vitamin B3) with meals. Should be taken only under medical supervision at doses > 1 g/day, because potentially serious side effects can occur, including liver inflammation and hyperglycemia.
To reduce risk of oxidation of blood cholesterol		
Vitamin C	1–2 g	Protects against fat oxidation; lowers tendency for platelet aggregation; lowers blood cholesterol. May reduce frequency and severity of angina.
Vitamin E and selenium	200–400 mg vitamin E; 200 μg selenium	Protects against LDL-cholesterol oxidation; lowers tendency for platelet aggregation. May reduce frequency and severity of angina.
To reduce elevated cholesterol and elevated blood pressure		
Calcium and magnesium	600 mg calcium; 300 mg magnesium. Can be taken as dolomite tablets	Calcium helps lower elevated cholesterol levels and may protect against atherosclerosis. Magnesium reduces cholesterol levels and raises HDLs; also reduces risk of dysrhythmias and reduces severity of angina.

Nutrient	Recommended Daily Dose	Comments
Omega-3 fatty acids	2–3 g of EPA and DHA as fish oil capsules	Reduces risk of atherosclerosis by reducing blood cholesterol and triglycerides, lowering blood pressure, and reducing tendency for platelet aggregation.
To improve myocardial energy metabolism		
Carnitine	1–2 g	Lowers total blood cholesterol while increasing HDLs. Reduces symptoms of angina by increasing efficiency of energy metabolism in the myocardium.
Coenzyme Q10	60–120 mg	Reduces symptoms of angina by increasing efficiency of energy metabolism in the myocardium. Supports heart function and cardiac output in hearts that are weakened by atherosclerosis.

References

Ascherio A. Metabolic and atherogenic effects of trans fatty acids. *J Intern Med.* 1995; 238:93.

Boushey CJ et al. A quantitative assessment of plasma homocysteine as a risk factor for vascular disease. Probable benefits of increasing folic acid intakes. *JAMA.* 1995; 274:1049.

Clarke R et al. Dietary lipids and blood cholesterol: quantitative meta-analysis of metabolic ward studies. *BMJ.* 1997; 314:112.

Connor SL, Connor WE. Are fish oils beneficial in the prevention and treatment of coronary artery disease? *Am J Clin Nutr.* 1997; 66:1020.

Daviglus ML et al. Fish consumption and 30-year risk of myocardial infarction. *N Engl J Med.* 1997; 336:1046.

Jandak J, Steiner M, Richardson PD. Alpha-tocopherol, an effective inhibitor of platelet adhesion. *Blood.* 1989; 73:141.

Kamikawa T et al. Effects of L-carnitine on exercise tolerance in patients with stable angina pectoris. *Japan Heart J.* 1984; 25:587.

Kok FJ et al. Decreased selenium levels in acute myocardial infarction. *JAMA.* 1989; 261:1161.

Langsjoen PH et al. Long-term efficacy and safety of coenzyme Q10 therapy for idiopathic dilated cardiomyopathy. *Am J Cardiol.* 1990; 65:521.

Luria MH. Effect of low-dose niacin on high density lipoprotein cholesterol and total cholesterol/high density lipoprotein cholesterol concentration. *Arch Intern Med.* 1988; 148:2493.

Peterson JC, Spence JD. Vitamins and progression of atherosclerosis in hyperhomocysteinemia. *Lancet.* 1998; 351:263.

Rapola JM et al. Effect of vitamin E and beta-carotene on the incidence of angina pectoris. *JAMA.* 1996; 275:693.

Reusser ME, McCarron DA. Micronutrient effects on blood pressure regulation. *Nutr Rev* 1994; 52:367.

Simon JA. Vitamin C and cardiovascular disease: a review. *J Am Coll Nutr.* 1992; 11:107.
Steinberg D. Antioxidant vitamins and coronary heart disease. *N Engl J Med.* 1993; 328:1487.
Stephens NG et al. Randomised controlled trial of vitamin E in patients with coronary disease. *Lancet.* 1996; 347:781.
Whelton PK, Klag MJ. Magnesium and blood pressure; Review of the epidemiologic and clinical trial experience. *Am J Cardiol.* 1989: 63:26G.

Dementia and Alzheimer's Disease

Diet

It is estimated that about one fourth of all dementias are caused by nutritional factors that are, at least partially, reversible. Deficiencies of several B vitamins—niacin (vitamin B3), vitamin B12, thiamin (vitamin B1), and folate—can cause dementia. Chronic heavy alcohol use can also produce dementia—large amounts of alcohol have a direct toxic effect on brain cells. Risk of developing multi-infarct dementia (and progression of the disorder in people already affected) can be reduced by following the dietary recommendations for prevention of high blood pressure and stroke (p. 163). People with Alzheimer's disease, because of their disability and poor diet habits, often develop nutritional deficiencies that can accelerate progression the disease.

Micronutrients

Nutrient	Recommended Daily Dose	Comments
Vitamin E and selenium	800–1200 mg vitamin E; 200 µg selenium	Antioxidants can protect against brain cell loss and may slow progression of Alzheimer disease.
L-Carnitine	1.5–2 g	May slow progression of Alzheimer's disease. Induces release of acetylcholine in the brain.
Choline and pantothenic acid	10–15 g (as high-quality lecithin); 100 mg pantothenic acid	May enhance synthesis and release of acetylcholine (Alzheimer's disease is characterized by loss of brain cells that produce acetylcholine).
Vitamin B12	1 mg/day via intramuscular injection for 1 week, then 1 mg/week by intramuscular injection	Deficiency in the brain may produce dementia in spite of normal blood levels. Absorption of dietary vitamin B12 is poor in many older people and in younger people with digestive disorders.
Vitamin B-complex	Containing ample amounts of thiamin (vitamin B1), niacin (vitamin B3), and folic acid	Vitamin B deficiencies can produce dementia, particularly in older people, those with chronic illnesses, and heavy alcohol users.

References

Blass JP et al. Thiamine and Alzheimer's disease: A pilot study. *Arch Neurol.* 1988; 45:833.
Bowman B. Acetyl-carnitine and Alzheimer's disease. *Nutr Rev.* 1992; 50:142.
Canty DJ, Zeisel SH. Lecithin and choline in human health and disease. *Nutr Rev.* 1994; 52:327.
Geldmacher DS, Whitehouse PJ. Evaluation of dementia. *N Engl J Med.* 1996; 335:330.
Lindenbaum J et al. Neuropsychiatric disorders caused by cobalamin deficiency in the absence of anemia or macrocytosis. *N Engl J Med.* 1988; 318:1720.
Perry IJ et al. Prospective study of serum total homocysteine concentration and risk of stroke in middle-aged British men. *Lancet.* 1995; 346:1395.
Sano M et al. A controlled trial of selegiline, alpha-tocopherol, or both as treatment for Alzheimer's disease. *N Engl J Med.* 1997; 336:1216.

Dental Caries

Diet

Sucrose is extremely cariogenic, while lactose (milk sugar) and fructose are less likely to cause cavities. Sticky, retentive forms of sugar are the most likely to promote cavities. Unlike sugars, fats and protein cannot be used by bacteria to produce acid. Moreover, fats can coat the teeth and form a protective layer, while proteins increase the buffering capacity of the saliva. Milk products or cheese rather than sugary foods at the end of meals can reduce acid formation and help prevent tooth decay. Optimal nutrition during childhood can encourage formation of thick, acid-resistant enamel. The teeth gradually form and calcify from birth through the teen years, and a generous dietary supply of protein, calcium, fluoride, and vitamins C and D are particularly important. Low-level fluoride supplementation has great benefits: adding trace amounts of fluoride to the water or salt supply can reduce the risk of caries in children by over two thirds. However, too much can actually impair enamel formation and cause weakened, discolored teeth. In areas where water is fluoridated, supplementation by other means, such as fluoride mouthwashes or tablets, is unnecessary. But in areas where the fluoride content of the water is very low or absent, supplements are beneficial. The best time to give a fluoride supplement is at bedtime, after teeth cleaning.

Micronutrients

Nutrient	Recommended Daily Dose	Comments
Fluoride	0.25 mg as drops during infancy; then 0.5–1 mg during childhood and adult years (see Table p. 45 ff.)	Only indicated if fluoride levels in drinking water are <0.7 mg/L. Can substantially toughen enamel against acid attack.
Multivitamin supplement for children	Should contain 10 µg vitamin D and 20–50 mg vitamin C	Vitamins D and C play important roles in tooth formation.
Calcium	200–400 mg	Particularly important from birth to 8 years during formation and mineralization of the teeth.

References

Horowitz HS. Commentary on and recommendations for the proper uses of fluoride. *J Public Health.* 1995; 55:57.
Mandel ID. Caries prevention: current strategies, new directions. *J Am Dent Assoc.* 1996; 127:1477.
Richmond VL. Thirty years of fluoridation: A review. *Am J Clin Nutr.* 1985; 41:129.

Depression

Diet

Low levels of certain brain neurotransmitters, including serotonin and norepinephrine, can produce depression. Synthesis of these neurotransmitters is dependent on both amino acid precursors and enzyme systems that contain essential micronutrients. Poor eating habits can contribute to depression by failing to provide the nutrients necessary for synthesis of important neurotransmitters. In turn, depression can then aggravate nutrient deficiencies by causing lack of appetite. Food sensitivities can interfere with brain chemistry and alter mood. People with mood swings, which fluctuate according to food habits, should investigate possible sensitivities and eliminate the offending foods. Although small amounts of caffeine can have mood-elevating properties, chronic high intake of coffee and black tea may aggravate anxiety and depression.

Micronutrients

Nutrient	Recommended Daily Dose	Comments
Phenylalanine	500 mg–3 g. Begin with 500 mg/day and increase gradually to dose which produces improvement	The amino acid precursor to norepinephrine, a mood-elevating neurotransmitter. Should be taken together with 50 mg vitamin B6.
Tryptophan	1–3 g	Can increase levels of brain serotonin, a mood-elevating neurotransmitter. Should be taken together with 50 mg vitamin B6.
Folic acid	0.8 mg–5 g	Can increase methylation reactions in the brain that may elevate mood. May increase response to serotonin-uptake inhibitors.
Vitamin B-complex	Containing at least 25 mg thiamin (vitamin B1), riboflavin (vitamin B2), niacin (vitamin B3), and vitamin B6	Marginal deficiencies of thiamin (vitamin B1), riboflavin (vitamin B2), niacin (vitamin B3), and vitamin B6 can produce depression.

Nutrient	Recommended Daily Dose	Comments
Vitamin B12	1 mg/week by intramuscular injection	Particularly effective in older people with fatigue and depression.

References

Adams PW et al. Effect of pyridoxine hydrochloride (vitamin B6) upon depression associated with oral contraception. *Lancet.* 1973; 1:897.

Alpert JE, Fava M. Nutrition and depression: the role of folate. *Nutr Rev.* 1997; 55:145.

Beckman V, Ludoph E. DL-phenylalanine as antidepressant. *Arzneimit Forschung.* 1978; 28:283.

Bottiglieri T. Folate, vitamin B12 and neuropsychiatric disorders. *Nutr Rev.* 1996; 54:382.

Brozek J. Psychological effects of thiamin restriction and deprivation in normal young men. *Am J Clin Nutr.* 1951; 5:104.

Crowdon JM. Neuro-transmitter precursors in the diet: their use in the treatment of brain diseases. In: Wurtman RJ, Wurtman JJ, eds. *Nutrition and the Brain, vol. 3.* New York: Raven Press; 1979.

Kravitz HM et al. Dietary supplements of phenylalanine and other amino acid precursors of brain neuroamines in the treatment of depressive disorders. *J Am Osteo Assoc.* 1984; 84:119.

Oren DA et al. A controlled trial of cyanocobalamin (vitamin B12) in the treatment of winter seasonal affective disorder. *J Affect Disord.* 1994; 32:197.

Reynolds EH et al. Methylation and mood. *Lancet.* 1984; 2:196.

Thomson J, Rankin H, Ashcroft GW, et al. The treatment of depression in general practice; a comparison of L-tryptophan, amitriptyline, and a combination of L-tryptophan and amitriptyline with placebo. *Psychol Med.* 1982; 12:741.

Diabetes Mellitus

Diet

The best way to prevent Type II diabetes is to avoid gaining weight: overweight people are four times more likely to develop Type II diabetes than people who maintain a normal body weight. Diabetics who are overweight can often reduce or eliminate their need for drugs and control their blood sugar by losing extra weight.
The glucose tolerance factor (GTF) is a naturally-occurring compound that helps regulate blood sugar. It is found in high amounts in brewer's yeast. Chromium is an essential component of GTF and diets deficient in chromium produce glucose intolerance. Diabetics who excrete glucose in their urine have increased urinary losses of minerals (such as magnesium, zinc, and chromium) due to an osmotic diuresis. Deficiencies of these important minerals further impair the ability to control blood glucose. Therefore, diabetic diets should emphasize foods rich in these minerals.
The best diet for most diabetics is one low in refined sugars and high in complex carbohydrates and fiber (which slow absorption of dietary sugars, reducing postprandial peaks in blood sugar). Foods like vegetables, fruits, legumes, and whole grains should be emphasized, and adopting a vegetarian or mostly vegetarian diet can be especially beneficial for a diabetic. To reduce elevated blood lipids and lower the risk of cardiovascular disease, saturated fat intake should be minimized and replaced by high-quality plant oils that supply the essential polyunsaturated fatty acids (PUFAs).

Micronutrients

Nutrient	Recommended Daily Dose	Comments
To enhance the action of insulin and help control blood glucose		
Vitamin E	800 mg; begin with 100 mg/day and gradually increase dose	Can enhance insulin sensitivity and reduce needs for oral hypoglycemics and/or insulin. Reduces platelet aggregation and risk of thrombosis.

Nutrient	Recommended Daily Dose	Comments
Chromium	200–400 μg chromium	As a component of GTF, helps control blood glucose and decrease need for insulin or hypoglycemic drugs. Can be taken together with 5–10 g brewer's yeast.
Vitamin C	1–2 g. Can be taken as a complex with bioflavonoids	Can help regulate blood glucose, strengthen small blood vessels, and reduce risk of early heart disease.
Prevention of mineral deficiencies which impair glucose tolerance		
Magnesium	400–600 mg	Magnesium deficiency is common in diabetes. Supplements may help control blood glucose and protect against cardiovascular disease.
Multimineral supplement	Balanced formula containing at least 15 mg zinc	Helps replenish urinary losses.
To treat diabetic neuropathy		
Gamma-linolenic acid (GLA)	As 2–4 g evening primrose oil (EPO)	Beneficial in treating neuropathy.
Myo-inositol	1–2 g	Beneficial in treating neuropathy.
Vitamin B-complex	High potency supplement containing at least 50 mg thiamin (vitamin B1) and vitamin B6	Neuropathic symptoms may respond to supplemental thiamin (vitamin B1) and vitamin B6.
To help control newly-diagnosed Type I diabetes		
Niacinamide	1–3 g; begin with 500 mg/day and increase dose gradually	Supplements in newly-diagnosed Type I diabetics can reduce insulin requirements and extend the time they can go before beginning insulin. Avoid nicotinic acid, another form of niacin (vitamin B3), which can be harmful in diabetics.

References

Caballero B. Vitamin E improves the action of insulin. *Nutr Rev.* 1993; 51:339.
Jain SK et al. The effect of modest vitamin E supplementation on lipid peroxidation products and other cardiovascular risk factors in diabetic patients. *Lipids.* 1996; 31:87.
Jamal GA et al. Gamma-linolenic acid in diabetic neuropathy. *Lancet.* 1986; 1:1098.
Lee NA, Reasner CA. Beneficial effects of chromium supplementation on serum triglyceride levels in NIDDM. *Diabetes Care.* 1994; 17:1449.
Offenbacher EG, Pi-Sunyer FX. Beneficial effects of chromium-rich yeast on glucose tolerance and blood lipids in elderly subjects. *Diabetes.* 1980; 29:919.
Paolisso G et al. Improved insulin response and action by chronic magnesium administration in aged NIDDM subjects. *Diabetes Care.* 1989; 12:265.
Paolisso G et al. Metabolic benefits deriving from chronic vitamin C supplementation in aged non-insulin dependent diabetics. *J Am Coll Nutr.* 1995; 14:387.
Pozzilli P et al. Meta-analysis of nicotinamide treatment in patients with recent-onset IDDM. *Diabetes Care.* 11996; 9:1357.
Rogers KS, Mohan C. Vitamin B6 metabolism and diabetes. *Biochem Med Metab Biol.* 1994; 52:10.
Salonen JT et al. Increased risk of non-insulin dependent diabetes mellitus at low plasma vitamin E concentrations: a four year follow up study in men. *BMJ.* 1995; 311:1124.
Salway JG et al. Effect of myo-inositol on peripheral-nerve function in diabetics. *Lancet.* 1978; 2:1281.
Ting HH et al. Vitamin C improves endothelium-dependent vasodilation in patients with non-insulin-dependent diabetes mellitus. *J Clin Invest.* 1996; 97:22.
Will JC, Byers T. Does diabetes mellitus increase the requirement for vitamin C? *Nutr Rev.* 1996; 54:193.

Eczema

Diet

A careful elimination diet can identify food sensitivities that trigger eczema. The most common offending foods are milk, eggs, fish, cheese, nuts, and food additives. Cold-pressed nut and seed oils are high in beneficial essential fatty acids important for skin health and should be consumed regularly. Disturbances in fatty acid metabolism in the skin can produce or aggravate eczema; impaired production of the omega-3 fatty acids from dietary linolenic acid (p. 79), as well as gamma-linolenic acid (GLA) from linoleic acid can increase inflammation in the skin.

Micronutrients

Nutrient	Recommended Daily Dose	Comments
Gamma-linolenic acid (GLA)	As 2–4 g evening primrose oil (EPO)	Can reduce inflammation and speed healing. Take with at least 100 International Units (IU) vitamin E.
Omega-3 fatty acids	1–1.5 g EPA from fish oil capsules	Skin salves containing EPA can also be applied to patches; take with at least 100 IU vitamin E.
Zinc	50 mg	Zinc-containing ointments applied to eczema can be beneficial.
Vitamin E	100–200 mg	Can help regulate skin proliferation and reduce symptoms.

References

Bjorneboe A et al. Effect of dietary supplementation with eicosapentaeonoic acid in the treatment of atopic dermatitis. *Br J Dermatol.* 1987; 117:463.
Endre L et al. Incidence of food allergy and zinc deficiency in children treated for atopic dermatitis. *Orv Hetail.* 1989; 130:2465.
Horrobin DF, Morse PF. Evening primrose oil and atopic eczema. *Lancet.* 1995; 345:260.
Mabin DC et al. Nutritional content of few foods diet in atopic dermatitis. *Arch Dis Child.* 1995; 73:208.
Olson PE et al. Oral vitamin E for refractory hand dermatitis. *Lancet.* 1994; 343:672.
Soyland E et al. Dietary supplementation with very long-chain n-3 fatty acids in patients with atopic dermatitis. A double-blind, multicentre study. *Br J Dermatol.* 1994; 130:757.

Epilepsy

Diet

In rare cases, food sensitivities can produce seizures in children with epilepsy who have a history of atopy. An elimination diet (p. 146) may identify food sensitivities that can contribute to epilepsy. The artificial sweetener aspartame may produce seizures in some children when consumed in high doses. Childhood seizures can be treated by a ketogenic diet—a specialized low-carbohydrate, high-fat diet that requires careful supervision. Alongside traditional anticonvulsants, micronutrients can play important adjuvant roles in seizure control.

Micronutrients

Nutrient	Recommended Daily Dose	Comments
Taurine	0.5–2 g	May reduce seizure severity and frequency.
Vitamin E and selenium	200–400 mg vitamin E; 100 μg selenium	When added to regular anticonvulsant therapy in children with epilepsy, can reduce seizure frequency.
Vitamin B6	50–250 mg	In some cases, seizures can be caused by inadequate production of the inhibitory neurotransmitter called gamma-aminobutyric acid (GABA). Vitamin B6 may stimulate production of GABA in the brain and reduce severity of seizures.
Multimineral supplement	Complete formula containing 300–400 mg magnesium and 10–20 mg manganese	Deficiency can cause seizures; epileptics often have low levels of body magnesium and manganese.

References

Allan RB. Nutritional aspects of epilepsy—a review of the potential of nutritional intervention in epilepsy. *Int Clin Nutr Rev.* 1983; 3:3.

Bernstein AL. Vitamin B6 in neurology. *Ann N Y Acad Sci.* 1990; 585:250.

Carl GF et al. Association of low blood manganese concentration with epilepsy. *Neurology* .1986; 36:1584.

Crowell GF, Roach ES. Pyridoxine-dependent seizures. *Am Fam Physician.* 1983; 27:183.

Durelli L, Tutani R. The current status of taurine in epilepsy. *Clin Neuropharmacol.* 1983; 6:37.

Egger J et al. Oligoantigenic diet treatment of children with epilepsy and migraine. *J Pediatr.* 1989; 114:51.

Goutieres F, Aicardi J. Atypical presentations of pyridoxine dependant seizures: a treatable cause of intractable epilepsy in infants. *Ann Neurol.* 1985; 17:117.

Raju GB et al. Randomized, double-blind, placebo-controlled, clinical trial of vitamin E as add-on therapy in uncontrolled epilepsy. *Epilepsia.* 1994; 35:368.

Ramaekers VT et al. Selenium deficiency triggering intractable seizures. *Neuropediatrics.* 1994; 25:217.

Takahashi R, Nakane Y. Clinical trial of taurine in epilepsy. In: Barbeau A, Huxtable RJ, eds. *Taurine and Neurological Disorders.* New York: Raven Press; 1978.

Fatigue

Diet

Along with adequate rest and regular exercise, a balanced and nutritious diet can help manage stress and avoid fatigue. Modern, affluent diets are typically high in energy, refined carbohydrate, salt, and saturated fat, but low in complex carbohydrates, fresh fruits, and vegetables. This dietary pattern often produces chronic, marginal deficiencies of several micronutrients—the B vitamins, magnesium, iron, and zinc—important to maintaining energy and fighting fatigue. Moreover, during periods of increased workload and stress, requirements for these micronutrients are higher. Emphasizing whole grains and lean sources of protein, along with fresh fruits and vegetables will provide ample amounts of the B vitamins and minerals needed to combat fatigue. Many people make the mistake of relying on large amounts of sugar and coffee during times of stress. Although they may supply short bursts of energy, too much caffeine and refined carbohydrate ultimately worsens chronic fatigue and produces headaches, irritability, and difficulty concentrating. Because control of blood glucose is more difficult during times of stress, it is important to minimize intake of refined carbohydrates, which may trigger periods of reactive hypoglycemia (p. 166).

Micronutrients

Nutrient	Recommended Daily Dose	Comments
Multimineral supplement	Balanced formula with 5–10 mg iron and 10–20 mg zinc	Especially prevalent in women and vegetarians, iron and zinc deficiencies can cause chronic fatigue.
Vitamin B-complex	Complete formula providing 10–25 mg thiamin (vitamin B1), riboflavin (vitamin B2), niacin (vitamin B3), and pantothenic acid, and 0.8 mg folic acid	Deficiencies of the B vitamins, because of their central role in energy production, produce fatigue. Requirements are higher during times of increased activity and energy expenditure.

Nutrient	Recommended Daily Dose	Comments
Vitamin C	250 mg	Marginal deficiency can produce fatigue and decrease alertness.
Vitamin B12	25–50 μg	Vitamin B12 deficiency produces anemia, fatigue, and depression, and is particularly common among the elderly.

References

Beard JL et al. Iron metabolism: a comprehensive review. *Nutr Rev.* 1996; 54:295.
Cousins RJ. Zinc. In: *Present Knowledge in Nutrition*. Ziegler EE, Filer LJ, eds. Washingon DC: ILSI Press; 1997: 293–306.
Middleman AB et al. Nutritional vitamin B12 deficiency and folate deficiency in an adolescent patient presenting with anemia, weight loss, and poor school performance. *J Adolesc Health.*1996; 19:76.

Fibrocystic Breast Disease

Diet

High-fat diets increase the risk of developing fibrocystic breast disease (FBD). In women with FBD, reducing the fat content of the diet (so that only 15–20% of calories come from fat) can reduce breast swelling and tenderness. Together with a low-fat diet, reducing or eliminating caffeine and theobromine (in black tea) can significantly improve symptoms.

Micronutrients

Nutrient	Recommended Daily Dose	Comments
Vitamin E	200–400 mg	Supplementation can reduce or eliminate symptoms in many women.
Gamma-linolenic acid (GLA)	As 2–4 g evening primrose oil (EPO)	May reduce lumpiness and tenderness, especially when symptoms are perimenstrual.
Vitamin A	5000–8000 μg	Supplementation can reduce swelling and tenderness. Large doses of vitamin A should be taken under medical supervision only.
Iodine	150–250 μg For severe cases, aqueous (diatomic) iodine (3 mg/day)	Can relieve pain and swelling, and reduce lumpiness. Kelp supplements are a rich source of iodine. Aqueous iodine should only be used under medical supervision.

References

Band PR et al. Treatment of benign breast disease with vitamin A. *Prev Med.* 1984; 13:549.

Boyd NF et al. Effect of a low-fat high-carbohydrate diet on symptoms of cyclical mastopathy. *Lancet.* 1988; 2:128.

Boyle CA et al. Caffeine consumption and fibrocystic breast disease: A case-control epidemiologic study. *J Natl Canc Inst.* 1984; 72:1015.

Ernster VL et al. Vitamin E and benign breast „disease“: a double-blind, randomized clinical trial. *Surgery.* 1985; 97:490.

London RF et al. The effect of vitamin E on mammary dysplasia: A double-blind study. *Obstet Gynecol.* 1985; 65:104.

Preece P et al. Evening primrose oil for mastalgia. In: Horrobin DF, ed. *Clinical Uses of Essential Fatty Acids.* London: Eden Press; 1982.

Food Sensitivities

Diet

Food sensitivities can produce a wide variety of symptoms (see Table below). Symptoms can be confined to the digestive tract, such as bloating, cramping, diarrhea, or the irritable bowel syndrome (p. 176). They can also occur in parts of the body far away from the digestive tract, such as the joints (arthritis), skin (swelling and hives), and brain (headache). Symptoms can occur immediately after eating the food, or may be delayed for hours. Food sensitivity can develop at any age, but is particularly common in infants and young children. About 7–10% of children exhibit food allergies during their growing years. Colic in babies may be caused by sensitivity to a food—a common allergen is the protein in cow's milk. Adults can also develop sensitivity reactions, particularly when stress, illness, or poor nutrition weakens the immune system.

The foods that are most commonly implicated in allergy and sensitivity reactions are shown in the Table below. Food allergies are often difficult to identify. Although many diagnostic tests have been tried, none is entirely satisfactory. A careful elimination diet remains the 'gold standard' test; if one of the eliminated foods was causing the reaction, improvement will occur. Foods must be eliminated for at least 5 days (and often for 2–4 weeks) to allow time for their adverse effects to completely disappear. If improvement occurs, the eliminated foods should be reintroduced one at a time to pinpoint the specific problem food. In order to discriminate between the effects of different foods, one food should be reintroduced about every 3 days. Keeping a food diary—recording the days and times foods are reintroduced and recording changes in symptoms—is essential. Foods that continue to be eaten during an elimination diet should be those least suspected of triggering symptoms. If there is uncertainty over which foods to eliminate and which to continue eating, the most practical approach is the *common-food elimination diet*. In this diet, only foods that are normally eaten more than twice a week are eliminated. More difficult is a *two-food diet*, such as the lamb-and-pear diet, where only two less commonly eaten foods—one supplying protein and fat, the other carbohydrate—are eaten. The remaining foods are then gradually reintroduced, one by one. More than three quarters of children with food allergies grow out of them. Reducing stress can reduce susceptibility to allergies. Nutritional deficiencies may increase vulnerability to food sensitivity reactions, which can gradually clear with proper diet and prudent nutritional supplementation

The following symptoms may be the result of food sensitivity:

- Acne
- Arthritis
- Asthma
- Abdominal pain and bloating
- Diarrhea
- Fatigue
- Swelling and fluid retention
- Headaches
- Nasal congestion
- Poor memory and concentration
- Repeated colds, sinus, and inner ear problems
- Itchy, watery eyes

Most common dietary triggers of food sensitivity reactions:

- Wheat, oats, corn
- Eggs
- Milk products
- Beef and pork
- Fish and shellfish
- Citrus fruits
- Peanuts
- Tomatoes
- Chocolate, tea, coffee
- Alcohol
- Food colorings, additives, and preservatives
- Monosodium glutamate (MSG)
- Sulfites—preservatives in fresh produce, salads, potatoes, wine
- Colorings—tartrazine (yellow dye)
- Benzoates
- Vanillin

Micronutrients

Nutrient	Recommended Daily Dose	Comments
Vitamin C	1–2 g	May increase breakdown of histamine produced as part of the allergic response, and thereby reduce symptoms.
Vitamin B6	50–100 mg	May reduce food sensitivities, particularly to additives such as MSG.
Omega-3 fatty acids	2–4 g as fish oil capsules	Reduces inflammation and may decrease symptoms.
Vitamin B12	50–100 μg	May reduce food sensitivity, particularly to sulfites.

References

Anonymous. Vitamin B12 confirmed as effective sulfite allergy blocker. *Allergy Observ.* 1987; 4:1.
Blok WL. Modulation of inflammation and cytokine production by dietary (n-3) fatty acids. *J Nutr.* 1996; 126:1515.
Bock SA, Atkins FM. Patterns of food hypersensitivity during sixteen years of double-blind, placebo-controlled food challenges. *J Pediatr.* 1990; 117:561.
Bruijnzeel-Koomen C et al. Adverse reactions to foods: European Academy of Allergology and Clinical Immunology Position Paper. *Allergy.* 1995; 50:623.
Terho EO, Savolainen J. Diagnosis of food hypersensitivity. *Eur J Clin Nutr.* 1996; 50:1.
Wüthrich B et al.: Food allergy. *Internist.* 1995; 36:1052.

Gallstones

Diet

Gallstones are found in about 10% of adults in the industrialized countries. Diet can have a major influence on the development of gallstones. High-fat diets, particularly saturated fat, and overconsumption of refined carbohydrates can stimulate gallstone development. Ample dietary fiber and moderate intake of alcohol decrease the risk. Being overweight sharply increases the risk of gallstones, while weight loss in obese persons can cause even chronic stones to dissolve and clear. In a person with gallstones, consumption of fatty foods or coffee can bring on painful gallbladder spasms. Also, food sensitivities are often an unrecognized trigger of gallbladder symptoms—eggs, pork, and onions are the most commonly implicated.

Micronutrients

Nutrient	Recommended Daily Dose	Comments
Taurine	1 g	Taurine is an important component of the bile and helps to keep cholesterol from precipitating in the gallbladder. Supplementation may reduce the risk of stone formation, especially in overweight women.
Vitamin E	400 mg	May help protect against the formation of gallstones, particularly when dietary fat intake is high. Supplementation can reduce symptoms and may stimulate gallstones to dissolve and clear.
Vitamin C	250 mg	Deficiency increases the risk of gallstones.

References

Maclure KM et al. Weight, diet, and the risk of symptomatic gallstones in middle-aged women. *N Engl J Med.* 1989; 321:563.

Saito T, Tanimura H. The preventive effect of vitamin E on gallstone formation. A study of the biliary lipids in patients with gallstones. *Arch Jap Chir.* 1987; 56:276.

Simon JA, Hudes ES. Serum ascorbic acid and gallbladder disease among US adults. *Arch Int Med* 2000; 160: 931–936.

Wang WY, Liaw KY. Effect of a taurine-supplemented diet on conjugated bile acids in biliary surgical patients. *Journal of Parenteral and Enteral Nutrition.* 1991; 15:294

Gingivitis and Periodontal Disease

Diet

A diet high in refined carbohydrates (especially sucrose) promotes periodontal disease. Frequent consumption of sugar increases plaque formation and increases the risk of gingivitis. Sugars also promote periodontal disease by reducing the ability of the white blood cells in the gums to destroy the pathogenic plaque bacteria. Sucrose is particularly destructive in sticky forms (like candy and baked goods) because they cling to the teeth for longer. Regular intake of foods rich in vitamin C, high-quality protein, and zinc can help maintain the integrity of the periodontal tissues.

Micronutrients

Nutrient	Recommended Daily Dose	Comments
Vitamin C	500 mg–1 g (best if taken together with a bioflavonoid complex)	Vitamin C may help heal inflamed gums and reduce gum bleeding. It also helps maintain the immune system to fight periodontal infection.
Folic acid	0,5–1 mg (can also be taken as a 0.1 % solution of folate mouthwash, rinsing with 1 tablespoon/twice daily)	Can be an effective treatment for periodontal disease; diseased gums may contain only low levels of folate.
Vitamin D and calcium	5–10 μg vitamin D and 600 mg calcium	Can help maintain the bones surrounding and supporting the teeth.

References

Fontana M. Vitamin C: clinical implications for oral health--a literature review. *Compendium* 1994; 15:916.
Leggott PJ. et al. The effect of controlled ascorbic acid depletion and supplementation on periodontal health. *J Periodontol* 1986; 57:480.
Pack ARC. Folate mouthwash: Effects on established gingivitis in periodontal patients. *J Clin Periodontol* 1984; 11:619.
Vogel RI. et al. The effects of megadoses of ascorbic acid on PMN chemotaxis and experimental gingivitis. *J Periodontol* 1986; 57:472.
Whalen JP. Krook L Periodontal disease as the early manifestation of osteoporosis. *Nutrition* 1996; 12:53–4
Wical KE. Brussee P. Effects of a calcium and vitamin D supplement on alveolar ridge resorption in immediate denture patients. *J Prosthet Dent* 1979; 41:4.

Glaucoma

Diet

Food sensitivities may increase intraocular pressure in people with glaucoma. Caffeine ingestion increases pressure in the eye, and excess dietary protein and trans-fatty acids (in hydrogenated fats) are associated with increased risk of glaucoma.

Micronutrients

Nutrient	Recommended Daily Dose	Comments
Vitamin C with bioflavonoids	1–2 g vitamin C with 200 mg rutin	Vitamin C, particularly together with rutin bioflavonoids, may help reduce eye pressure in glaucoma.
Thiamin (vitamin B1)	25 mg	Thiamin deficiency may contribute to the development of glaucoma.
Multimineral supplement	Should contain zinc (10–20 mg) and chromium (200 μg)	Reduced zinc and chromium intake are associated with higher eye pressures, and deficiencies may aggravate glaucoma.

References

Higginbotham EJ. et al. The effect of caffeine on intraocular pressure in glaucoma patients. *Ophthalmology* 1989; 96:624.
Virno M. et al. Oral treatment of glaucoma with vitamin C. *Eye Ear Nose Throat Month* 1967; 46:1502.

Heavy Metal Intoxication

Toxic metals (lead, cadmium, mercury, aluminum) are naturally present in only trace quantities in the earth's crust. Modern industry has extracted these metals from the earth, concentrated them in various forms, and then dispersed them throughout the environment. Over the past century, our food, water, and air have become tainted with these metals. Once ingested, they tend to accumulate in the body over time—depositing in the skeleton, liver, and kidneys. Today, the average city-dweller has a body toxic metal burden 500–1000 times greater than that of people living in the pre-industrial age. Even at low-levels of exposure, toxic metals are potent poisons. They are thought to contribute to many modern ailments, including cancer, high blood pressure, and learning impairments in children.

Lead

The main sources of lead pollution are:

- Auto exhaust (food grown near cities, industry, or busy roads)
- House paint (many older paints are very high in lead), house dust
- Lead plumbing (lead leaches into drinking water)
- Industrial smoke from coal burning
- Canned foods (some canning processes use lead sealants)
- Milk from animals grazing on grass containing traces of lead
- Pottery and glassware with lead-containing glaze or paint
- Car batteries, lead-shot, certain hair dyes, inks
- Cigarette smoke

The potential effects of low-level lead exposure include:

- Learning problems, reduced intelligence, and hyperactivity in children (exposure to lead during pregnancy can lead to permanent mental impairment of the infant)
- Headache, fatigue, irritability
- Anorexia and diarrhea
- Depression, insomnia
- May increase risk of cancer
- May increase risk of high blood pressure and heart disease

Laboratory Measurement of Status

Measure	Values	Comment
Blood lead level	Levels > 200 μg/L indicate elevated tissue levels and toxicity.	Blood levels are a relatively insensitive index of chronic exposure, as the majority of body lead is deposited in the skeleton.
Hair lead level	Levels > 15 μg/g may indicate elevated tissue levels.	Hair analysis is a reliable measure of tissue levels.
Zinc protoporphyrin in red blood cells	Levels > 40 μmol/mol heme may indicate elevated tissue levels.	Lead interferes with normal synthesis of hemoglobin. Elevated levels may also be caused by iron deficiency.

Aluminum

The main sources of aluminum are:

- Cookware (avoid aluminum pots and pans, particularly when cooking vegetables, fruit, and other acidic foods that leach large amounts of aluminum from cookware), household and industrial utensils
- Aluminum-containing antacids
- Aluminum cans
- Deodorants, antiperspirants, cosmetics, toothpastes
- Refined white flour (aluminum-containing compounds are often used to bleach the flour)
- Anticlumping additives to salt and spices, baking powder

The potential effects of low-level aluminum exposure include:

- Disorders of the central nervous system: impaired memory, may increase risk of Alzheimer's disease
- Impaired bone metabolism (may weaken bones and increase risk of osteoporosis)
- Liver and kidney toxicity
- May accumulate in joints and trigger arthritis

Laboratory Measurement of Status

Measure	Values	Comment
Hair aluminum level	Normal levels are 3–40 μg/g.	Hair analysis is a reliable measure of tissue levels.

Mercury

The main sources of mercury are:

- Amalgam dental fillings
- Pesticides, fungicides, industrial waste
- Fish and shellfish from contaminated waters (they tend to concentrate mercury)

The potential effects of low-level mercury exposure include:

- Mental impairment, difficulty concentrating, headache
- Nerve damage that mimics multiple sclerosis
- If babies are exposed in utero: cerebral palsy, mental retardation, birth defects
- Skin rash
- Increased risk of cancer

Laboratory Measurement of Status

Measure	Values	Comment
Urinary mercury excretion	Levels > 1.5 μg/day indicate elevated tissue levels.	Urinary excretion is a good index of total body burden.
Hair mercury level	Levels > 3.0 μg/g may indicate elevated tissue levels.	Hair analysis is a reliable measure of tissue levels.

Cadmium

The main sources of cadmium are:

- Metal coatings (cadmium is an anticorrosive) on metal pails, cans, refrigerator ice trays, water tanks
- Cigarette smoke (a concentrated source, containing about 20 μg per cigarette). Smokers generally have body levels five times as high as nonsmokers

- Insecticides
- Certain foods: instant coffee, canned foods, gelatine, some cola drinks, kidneys from animals given cadmium-containing worm-killing drugs
- Fish and shellfish from contaminated waters
- Pigments (especially red and yellow colors)

The effects of low-level exposure include:

- May increase risk of high blood pressure
- May increase risk of cancer
- May impair immune function

Laboratory Measurement of Status

Measure	Values	Comment
Hair cadmium levels	Levels $> 1.6\,\mu g/g$ hair may indicate elevated tissue levels.	Hair analysis is a reliable measure of tissue levels and is superior to blood levels as an index of long-term exposure.

Diet

- *Water*
  Contamination from plumbing can be minimized by installing new plumbing if the old pipes are corroded, or contain lead or galvanized coatings rich in cadmium. 'Soft' water leaches more heavy metals from pipes than 'hard' water (another benefit of hard water is that it is richer in calcium and magnesium). High-quality water filters can minimize intake from drinking water. Do not take water for cooking and drinking from the hot-water tap if the plumbing is old (hot water leaches more metals from pipes). Flush the water pipes out before drawing water for drinking, especially in the morning or after periods when the pipes have not been used and water has stood in them.
- *Food*
  Avoid food and wine grown in gardens or vineyards located near heavily-trafficked roads. Avoid produce that is displayed outdoors near heavily-trafficked roads. Avoid cooking in aluminum pots and pans, and substitute stainless steel or enamel pots. Avoid canned foods, particularly acidic foods like fruits and tomatoes. Wipe the lip of newly-opened wine bottles carefully to remove lead traces from the foil surrounding the cork.

Micronutrients

To speed elimination of toxic metals from the body and prevent accumulation:

Nutrient	Recommended Daily Dose	Comments
Vitamin E and selenium	200–400 mg vitamin E; 200 μg selenium	Helps reduce the adverse effects of lead and mercury.
Vitamin C	250 mg	May enhance excretion of toxic metals, protects against oxidative damage.
Calcium and magnesium	400 mg calcium; 200 mg magnesium	Reduces lead and cadmium absorption.
Zinc	15–30 mg	May reduce absorption of cadmium; may enhance excretion of lead.

References

Baghurst PA. et al. Environmental lead exposure and children's intelligence at the age of seven years. *N Engl J Med* 1992; 327:1279.
Cuvin-Aralar ML. Furness RW. Mercury and selenium interaction: a review. *Ecotoxicol Environ Safety* 1991; 21:348.
Dhawan M. et al. Preventive and therapeutic role of vitamin E in chronic plumbism. *Biomed Environ Sci* 1989; 2:335.
Doll R. Review: Alzheimer's disease and environmental aluminum. *Age Ageing* 1993; 22:138.
Ehle AL. Mckee DC. Neuropsychological effect of lead in occupationally exposed workers: a critical review. *Crit Rev Toxicol* 1990; 20:237.
Exley C. et al. Aluminum toxicokinetics. *J Toxicol Environ Health* 1996; 48:569.
Flora SJS. Tandon SK. Adjuvants for therapeutic chelating drugs in lead intoxication. Trace Elem Electrol 1995; 12:131.
Houston DK. Does vitamin C protect against lead toxity? *Nutr Rev* 2000; 58:73–75.
Nakagawa H. Nishijo M. Environmental cadmium exposure, hypertension, and cardiovascular risk. *J Cardiovasc Risk* 1996; 3:11.
Pleva J. Dental mercury: a public health hazard. *Rev Environ Health* 1994; 10:1.
Ratcliffe HE. et al. Human exposure to mercury: a critical assessment of the evidence of adverse health effects. *J Toxicol Environ Health* 1996; 49:221.
Robards K. Worsfold P. Cadmium: toxicology and analysis: A review. *Analyst* 1991; 116:549.
Singh B. et al. Impact of lead pollution on the status of the other trace elements in blood and alterations in hepatic functions. *Biol Trace Elem Res* 1994; 40:21.
Weiss ST. et al. The relationship of blood lead to blood pressure in a longitudinal study of working men. *Am J Epidemiol* 1986; 123:800.

Herpes Simplex

Diet

For people with herpes, optimal nutrition and stress reduction may help reduce the frequency and severity of infections (see p. 168). The dietary ratio of two amino acids may influence herpes infections. High intakes of arginine promote growth of the virus (the herpes virus requires arginine for growth), while higher intakes of lysine may inhibit growth, mainly by reducing the amount of arginine available to the virus. Therefore, a lysine-rich, arginine-poor diet can help reduce recurrence and severity of herpes infections. Foods that have a particularly high ratio of arginine/lysine, and that should generally be avoided by people with recurrent herpes include:

- Nuts (particularly almonds, hazelnuts, cashews, and peanuts)
- Chocolate
- Seeds and certain grains (wheat, oats)
- Raisins, gelatine

Micronutrients

Nutrient	Recommended Daily Dose	Comments
Lysine	500 mg to help prevent recurrences, 2–4 g during active infection	Along with supplemental lysine, reduce intake of arginine-rich foods. May reduce severity and frequency of outbreaks.
Vitamin C	250–500 mg to help prevent recurrences 1 g to help treat active infections	Has antiviral action and may help reduce the severity and shorten the duration of recurrent infections.
Vitamin E	Apply topically to lesions (a soft gel capsule containing 100–400 mg can be punctured and the contents applied to blisters several times a day)	May help reduce pain and enhance healing.
Zinc	15–30 mg to help prevent recurrences, 60–100 mg during active infection. Can also be applied topically in zinc-containing creams or lotions	Has antiviral action and may help reduce the severity and shorten the duration of recurrent infections.

References

Eby G. Use of topical zinc to prevent recurrent herpes simplex infection: Review of literature and suggested protocols. *Med Hypotheses.* 1985; 17:157.
Griffith RS et al. Success of L-lysine therapy in frequently recurrent herpes simplex infection. *Dermatologica.* 1987; 175:183.
Terezhalmy GT et al. The use of water-soluble bioflavonoid-ascorbic acid complex in the treatment of recurrent herpes labialis. *Oral Surg.* 1978; 45:56.

Hyperactivity

Diet

Breakfast is the crucial meal for children with hyperactivity (attention deficit hyperactivity disorder, ADHD). Skipping breakfast can cause drops in blood sugar that can trigger restlessness and irritability. Breakfasts high in protein and calcium have a calming influence in many children and improve learning capability in ADHD. Children may be sensitive to high amounts of phosphates present in certain foods, including sausages, processed foods, milk products, and soft drinks. Food sensitivities can produce or aggravate ADHD. Artificial food colors and flavors, as well as foods containing natural salicylates, may trigger ADHD.

Foods to be avoided in children with ADHD:

- All foods containing artificial colors, sweeteners, and flavors
- Foods containing natural salicylates:

almonds	apple cider and vinegar	apricots	blackberries
cherries	cloves	cucumbers	pickles
grapes	raisins	mint flavors	nectarines
oranges	peaches	plums	strawberries
tomatoes	wine	vinegar	raspberries

Micronutrients

Nutrient	Recommended Daily Dose	Comments
Vitamin B-complex	Complete formula emphasizing thiamin (vitamin B1) and vitamin B6	May produce improvement in behavior and attention.
Essential PUFAs	Omega-3 fatty acids (1–2 g EPA as fish oil capsules) and Gamma-linolenic acid (GLA) as 1–2 g evening primrose oil (EPO)	PUFA metabolism may be abnormal in children with ADHD, and deficiencies of omega-3 and omega-6 fatty acids are found in many children with ADHD.
Multimineral supplement	Balanced supplement containing ample amounts of zinc and magnesium	Deficiencies of magnesium and zinc may aggravate ADHD.

References

Egger J et al. Controlled trial of oligoantigenic treatment in the hyperkinetic syndrome. *Lancet.* 1985; 1:540.
Feingold BF. *Why Your Child is Hyperactive.* New York: Random House; 1974.
Schulte-Korne G et al. Effect of an oligo-antigen diet on the behavior of hyperkinetic children. *Kinder Jugendpsychiatr.* 1996; 24:176.
Stevens LJ et al. Essential fatty acid metabolism in boys with attention-deficit hyperactivity disorder. *Am J Clin Nutr.* 1995; 62:761.

Hypertension and Stroke

Diet

The major dietary risk factors for hypertension and stroke are:

- *Overweight*
  Obesity is commonly associated with high blood pressure. Hypertensives who are overweight and who lose weight often experience significant reductions in blood pressure.
- *Low intake of PUFAs*
  Especially when combined with a high intake of saturated fat, low intake of essential PUFAs can increase risk of high blood pressure.
- *Salt*
  Although for most people sodium in the diet plays only a minor role in determining blood pressure, some individuals are very sensitive to sodium in the diet. People who have a family history of hypertension, are black, or are older than 55 are most likely to be sodium-sensitive. In these individuals, a diet high in sodium elevates blood pressure. About one third of people with high hypertension can lower their blood pressure significantly by limiting sodium intake, most of which comes from salt added to processed foods, such as canned soups and salty snacks.
- *Potassium*
  High sodium intake is a much stronger risk factor when combined with low intakes of potassium. People with low intakes of potassium are nearly five times more likely to die from stroke than those with higher intakes. Achieving a balanced intake of sodium/potassium should be a goal for people with hypertension and for people at risk of developing the disease. High-potassium/low-sodium foods, like potatoes, green vegetables, orange juice, apricots, and bananas, can be beneficial.
- *Calcium*
  Low dietary intake of calcium is associated with a higher risk of hypertension, and increasing intake of calcium (from supplements or calcium-rich foods like low-fat milk products, sesame seeds, or dark green leafy vegetables) can reduce blood pressure in people who are hypertensive.
- *Alcohol*
  Chronic high alcohol intake (more than two to three drinks per day) increases the risk of hypertension and stroke. People who drink reg-

ularly and have high blood pressure can often see a significant drop in blood pressure after a few days of abstention.

- *Antioxidants and other food components*
  High intake of dietary antioxidants from regular consumption of fruits and vegetables (particularly carrots and spinach) protects against high blood pressure, and can cut the risk of stroke in half. Garlic has blood pressure lowering effects and should be eaten regularly by people with hypertension.

Micronutrients

Nutrient	Recommended Daily Dose	Comments
For treatment of hypertension		
Calcium and magnesium	1.5 g calcium and 600 mg magnesium; can be taken as dolomite tablets	Dietary deficiencies of calcium and/or magnesium increase blood pressure; supplements can produce vasodilation and lower blood pressure.
Coenzyme Q10	60–120 mg	Lowers blood pressure in many people with hypertension.
Omega-3 fatty acids	2–3 g of EPA and DHA as fish oil capsules	Reduces blood pressure in hypertension.
Taurine	3 g	Lowers blood pressure in many people with hypertension.
In addition to the above, for prevention of stroke		
Vitamin B-complex	Should contain 0.8–1 mg folic acid, 25–50 mg vitamin B6 as part of a balanced formula	Reduces blood homocysteine levels and lowers risk of platelet aggregation, thereby reducing risk of stroke.
Vitamin E and selenium	200 mg vitamin E; 200 μg selenium	Reduces platelet aggregation and helps protect against stroke in people with hypertension.

References

Allender PS et al. Dietary calcium and blood pressure: a meta-analysis of the randomized clinical trials. *Ann Intern Med.* 1996; 124:825.

Bonaa KH et al. Effect of EPA and DHA on blood pressure in hypertension. *N Engl J Med.* 1990; 322:795.

Bronner LL et al. Primary prevention of stroke. *N Engl J Med.* 1995; 333:1392.

Greenberg S, Frishman WH. Coenzyme Q10: a new drug for cardiovascular disease. *J Clin Pharmacol.* 1990; 30:596–608.

Manson JE, Stampfer MJ, Willett WC et al. Antioxidant vitamin consumption and incidence of stroke in women. *Circulation.* 1993; 87:678.

Morimoto A et al. Sodium sensitivity and cardiovascular events in patients with essential hypertension. *Lancet.* 1997; 350:1734.

Hypoglycemia (reactive)

Diet

A diet plan to reduce reactive hypoglycemia should include:

- Avoiding simple sugars and refined carbohydrates (such as white flour and white rice). These stimulate rapid rises in blood glucose that trigger oversecretion of insulin.
- Substituting foods high in complex carbohydrates and fiber (which slow absorption of dietary sugars, reducing glycemic peaks during meals) like vegetables, legumes, oats, and whole grains.
- Eating five to six small meals spaced throughout the day to provide a constant source of energy to maintain blood sugar. Each meal should include foods containing high-quality protein and moderate amounts of cold-pressed plant oils.
- Avoiding large amounts of alcohol and coffee, which can exacerbate reactive hypoglycemia.
- Eating foods that have a low to moderate glycemic index and avoiding foods with a very high index. The glycemic index is a measure of a food's potential to rapidly elevate blood glucose. In people who are vulnerable to reactive hypoglycemia, these foods may stimulate insulin oversecretion.

The glycemic index of selected foods:

Very high	*High*	*Moderate*	*Low*	*Very Low*
Honey	Whole wheat bread	Buckwheat	Pasta	Nuts
Potatoes	Brown rice	Oat flakes	Sweet potatoes	Soybeans
Carrots	Raisins	Sweet corn	Navy beans	Kidney beans
Cornflakes	Banana	Green peas	Oranges	Lentils
White bread			Fructose	
White rice			Apples	
Beer			Milk and yogurt	
Sucrose			Tomatoes	

Micronutrients

Nutrient	Recommended Daily Dose	Comments
Chromium	200–400 μg	May help regulate blood glucose levels.
Multimineral supplement	Balanced supplement with 200 mg magnesium, 20 mg zinc, and 5 mg manganese	Deficiencies of zinc, magnesium, and manganese increase risk of reactive hypoglycemia.

References

Anderson RA et al. Effects of supplemental chromium on patients with symptoms of reactive hypoglycemia. *Metabolism.* 1987; 35:351.
Gorman JM et al. Hypoglycemia and panic attacks. *Am J Psychiatry.* 1984; 141:101.
Hofeldt FD. Reactive hypoglycemia. *Endocrinol Metab Clin North Am.* 1989; 18:185.
Stebbing JB et al. Reactive hypoglycaemia and magnesium. *Magnesium Bull.* 1982; 4:131.

Infection

Diet

Optimal micronutrition plays a central role in maintaining the health of the epithelial tissues as a barrier to potential pathogens. Also, both the humoral and cellular components of the immune system are dependent on nutrition. The immune system is weakened by even marginal deficiencies of vitamins A, C, E, B6, B12, and folate, as well as lack of the minerals iron, zinc, manganese, copper, or selenium. Deficiencies of micronutrients can impair production of new white cells and their activation and activity against foreign substances and cells. Certain micronutrients (such as vitamins E, C, and B6, and selenium and zinc) can boost the immune system, enhance white cell activity and function, and increase resistance to infection. Diets high in refined carbohydrate and saturated fat can weaken the immune system. Regular heavy alcohol intake also impairs function of the immune system and increases the risk of infection. To maintain immune strength, the diet should emphasize lean meats and low-fat milk products, whole grains, and fresh fruits and vegetables.

Micronutrients

Nutrient	Recommended Daily Dose	Comments
Vitamin A	3000–6000 μg to help prevent infection. Up to 30 000 μg to help treat active infection. Can be taken as beta-carotene	Enhances immune system function. Deficiency sharply increases risk of infection. Maintains the health of the skin and mucosal barriers to pathogens.
Vitamin C	100–500 mg to help prevent infection. Up to 5 g to help treat active infection	Enhances immune cell function. May be effective in reducing severity of infections, particularly those caused by viruses.
Vitamin E	100–200 mg to help prevent infection	Enhances immune cell function and may increase resistance to infection, particularly among the elderly.

Nutrient	Recommended Daily Dose	Comments
Vitamin B6	25–50 mg to help prevent infection. 250–500 mg to help treat active infection	Enhances immune cell function and may increase resistance to infection.
Zinc	10–20 mg to help prevent infection. Up to 100 mg to help treat active infection	Enhances immune cell function and may increase resistance to infection.
Selenium	100 µg to help prevent infection. 200–400 µg to help treat active infection	Deficiency increases risk and severity of infections, particularly those caused by viruses.

References

Anderson R. The immunostimulatory, anti-inflammatory and anti-allergic properties of ascorbate. *Adv Nutr Res.* 1984; 6:19.

Bendich A. Carotenoids and the immune response. *J Nutr.* 1989; 119:112.

Bogden JD et al. Effects of one year of supplementation with zinc and other micronutrients on cellular immunity in the elderly. *J Nutr.* 1990; 3:214.

Calder PC. Glutamine and the immune system. *Clin Nutr.* 1994; 13:2.

Dallman PR. Iron deficiency and the immune response. *Am J Clin Nutr.* 1987; 46:329.

Grimble RF. Effect of antioxidative vitamins on immune function with clinical applications. *Int J Vitam Nutr Res.* 1997; 67:312.

Jeng KCG et al. Supplementation with vitamins C and E enhances cytokine production by peripheral blood mononuclear cells in healthy adults. *Am J Clin Nutr.* 1996; 64:960.

Kiremidjian-Schumacher L, Stotzky G. Selenium and immune responses. *Environmental Research.* 1987; 42:277.

Lesourd BM et al. The role of nutrition in immunity in the aged. *Nutr Rev.* 1998; 56:113.

Meydani SN, Beharka AA. Recent developments in vitamin E and immune response. *Nutr Rev.* 1998; 56:49.

Rall LC, Meydani SN. Vitamin B6 and immune competence. *Nutr Rev.* 1993; 51:217.

Semba RD. The role of vitamin A and related retinoids in immune function. *Nutr Rev.* 1998; 56:38.

Solomons NW. Mild zinc deficiency produces an imbalance between cell-mediated and humoral immunity. *Nutr Rev.* 1998; 56:27.

Talbott MC et al. Pyridoxine supplementation: Effect on lymphocyte responses in elderly persons. *Am J Clin Nutr.* 1987; 46:659.

Infertility

Females

Diet

In women, being overweight or underweight can impair fertility. Excessive thinness from vigorous dieting or strenuous exercise is a common cause of infertility in women in the industrialized countries. In women who are underweight and have body fat content lower than 16–18% of body weight (women normally have about 25% body fat), ovarian production of estrogen is reduced. This can impair ovulation, interrupt the menstrual cycle, and produce infertility. On the other hand, too much body fat can also interfere with ovulation and cause infertility. About one in 10 overweight women have irregular menstrual cycles. Weight loss in overweight, infertile women can cause a return of ovulation and fertility. High intakes of alcohol and caffeine may also reduce fertility in women. Women trying to conceive should limit their alcohol intake to less than two glasses of wine or beer per day, and minimize their coffee intake. Deficiencies of vitamins E, B12, and folate, as well as iron and zinc, can reduce fertility. A high body burden of toxic metals (such as lead, mercury, and cadmium) may also impair fertility.

Micronutrients

Nutrient	Recommended Daily Dose	Comments
Multimineral supplement	Balanced formula containing 10–20 mg zinc and 10 mg iron	Deficiencies of iron or zinc may impair fertility.
Vitamin B-complex	Balanced supplement containing 0.4–0.8 mg folic acid and 2–5 μg vitamin B12	Deficiencies of folate and vitamin B12 may impair fertility.

Males

Diet

In men, poor nutrition—a diet high in refined carbohydrates, saturated fat, and processed foods, and low in important micronutrients—may reduce sperm count and motility. To help increase sperm quality, the diet should emphasize high-quality protein, whole grains, and fresh fruits and vegetables. Heavy alcohol drinking (more than 3 drinks per day) can impair fertility. Overweight men are more likely to have low testosterone levels and lower sperm count.

Micronutrients

Nutrient	Recommended Daily dose	Comments
Vitamin C	500 mg–1 g	Reduces abnormal clumping of sperm that can cause infertility; may improve sperm motility.
Arginine	2–4 g	Can improve sperm count and quality.
Zinc	60 mg	Essential for sperm production and synthesis of testosterone. Supplementation may improve sperm counts.
Multimineral supplement	Balanced supplement with 50–100 μg selenium and 100–200 μg chromium	Deficiencies of selenium and chromium can reduce sperm count.

References

Calloway DH. Nutrition and reproductive function of man. *Nutr Abstr Rev-Rev Clin Nutr.* 1983; 53:361.
Dawson EB et al. Effect of ascorbic acid on male fertility. *Ann N Y Acad Sci.* 1987; 498:312.
Keen CL, Bendich A, Wilhite CC, eds. Maternal Nutrition and Pregnancy Outcome. *Ann N Y Acad Sci.* 1993; 678:1–372.
Piesse J. Zinc and human male infertility. *Int Clin Nutr Rev* 1983; 3:4.
Rushton DH. Ferritin and fertility. *Lancet.* 1991; 337:1554.
Schachter A et al. Treatment of oligospermia with the amino acid arginine. *J Urol.* 1973; 110:311.
Shoupe D. Effect of body weight on reproductive function. In: Mishell DR, Darajan V, Lobo R, eds. *Infertility, Contraception and Reproductive Endocrinology*. Boston: Blackwell; 1991.
Takihara H et al. Zinc sulfate therapy for infertile males with or without varicocelectomy. *Urology.* 1987; 29:638.

Inflammatory Bowel Disease: Ulcerative Colitis and Crohn's Disease

Diet

People with active Inflammatory Bowel Disease (IBD) often become severely malnourished due to loss of appetite and malabsorption of nutrients. Dietary deficiencies are common and nutritional status must be carefully monitored. Body levels of minerals (calcium, magnesium, zinc, and iron) are often low in people with IBD. People with Crohn's disease affecting the ileum absorb vitamin B12 poorly, and may need periodic B12 injections. In many people, a high-fiber, low-refined carbohydrate diet reduces severity and recurrences in IBD, and, if followed long-term, reduces need for hospital care and intestinal surgery. Food sensitivities may aggravate IBD, and identification and avoidance of offending foods may increase the chances of remission. During acute exacerbations of Crohn's disease, enteral nutrition using protein hydrolysate diets is effective, and may help avoid steroid therapy.

Micronutrients

Nutrient	Recommended Daily Dose	Comments
Omega-3 fatty acids	2.5–3 g EPA (as fish oil capsules)	Can reduce extent and severity of inflammation and may improve symptoms.
Vitamin E	400 mg	Can reduce bowel inflammation and aid healing of the intestine.
L-Glutamine	1–1.5 g	Glutamine promotes healing of the intestinal mucosa.
Zinc	30–60 mg	Can promote healing of intestine.
Multivitamin/mineral supplement	A balanced supplement containing at least 0.8 mg folate and 50 μg vitamin B12, as well as magnesium, zinc, and iron	Malabsorption is common during active IBD. Folic acid and vitamin B12 may help protect against development of colon cancer in chronic ulcerative colitis.

References

Belluzzi A et al. Effect of an enteric-coated fish oil preparation on relapses in Crohn's disease. *N Engl J Med.* 1996; 334:1557.
Dronfield MW et al. Zinc in ulcerative colitis; a therapeutic trial and report on plasma levels. *Gut.* 1977; 18:33.
Greenfield SM et al. A randomized controlled study of evening primrose oil and fish oil in ulcerative colitis. *Aliment Pharmacol Ther.* 1993; 7:159.
Griffiths AM et al. Meta-analysis of enteral nutrition as a primary treatment of active Crohn's disease. *Gastroenterol.* 1995; 108:1056.
Harries AD, Heatley RV. Nutritional disturbances in Crohn's disease. *Postgrad Med J.* 1983; 50:690.
Heaton KW et al. Treatment of Crohn's disease with an unrefined- carbohydrate, fibre-rich diet. *BMJ.* 1979; 2:764.
Hendricks KM, Walker WA. Zinc deficiency in inflammatory bowel disease. *Nutr Rev.* 1988; 46:401.
Lashner BA et al. Effect of folate supplementation on the incidence of dysplasia and cancer in chronic ulcerative colitis: A case controlled study. *Gastroenterol.* 1989; 97:255.

Insomnia

Diet

The amino acid tryptophan is a precursor for brain synthesis of serotonin, a sleep-inducing neurotransmitter. Eating foods rich in tryptophan as a late-evening snack (together with a small amount of carbohydrate) can improve sleep quality. Carbohydrates stimulate production of insulin, and insulin enhances uptake of tryptophan into the brain.
Although alcohol has a sedative effect that can hasten sleep onset, heavy alcohol intake often produces light, unsettled sleep, and increases nighttime awakening. A good bedtime drink is a glass of warm milk. Milk is rich in tryptophan and calcium, both of which have a calming effect and may improve sleep quality. Avoid coffee, tea, or cola drinks within 6 hours of bedtime, and minimize consumption during the day. Low nighttime blood sugar levels can cause frequent or early awakening, and may be a sign of reactive hypoglycemia (p. 166).

Foods with a high tryptophan/protein ratio:

- Walnuts
- Soybeans and soy products
- Bananas
- Milk and milk products
- Eggs
- Fish

Micronutrients

Nutrient	Recommended Daily Dose	Comments
Tryptophan	1–3 g, 30 minutes before bedtime	Helps to improve sleep patterns.
Melatonin	1–5 mg, 30–60 minutes before bedtime	Particularly effective in people over 50 years of age with chronic insomnia.
Niacinamide	1 g, 30 minutes before bed	Helps to hasten onset of sleep and may improve quality of sleep.

References

Garfinkel D et al. Improvement of sleep quality in elderly people by controlled release melatonin. *Lancet.* 1995; 346:541.

Hartman E, Spinweber CL. Sleep induced by L-tryptophan: Effect of dosages within the normal dietary intake. *J Nerv Ment Dis.* 1979; 167:497.

Hofeldt FD. Reactive hypoglycemia. *Endocrinol Metab Clin North Am.* 1989; 18:185.

Möhler H et al. Nicotinamide is a brain constituent with benzodiazepine-like actions. *Nature* 1979; 278:563–565.

Wyatt RJ et al. Effects of L-tryptophan (a natural sedative) on human sleep. *Lancet.* 1970; 1:842.

Young SN. Behavioral effects of dietary neurotransmitter precursors: basic and clinical aspects. *Neurosci Biobehav Rev.* 1996; 20:313.

Irritable Bowel Syndrome

Diet

There is no single cause of irritable bowel syndrome (IBS). Many factors can trigger the disease, including:

- Diets too low or too high in fiber may worsen symptoms. Obtaining moderate amounts of dietary fiber by eating whole grains, vegetables, fruits, and legumes can be beneficial.
- Sensitivity to sugars. The disorder may be triggered by ingestion of sucrose, fructose, or sorbitol (a sugar alcohol used in low-calorie candy and chewing gum).
- Lactose intolerance. Levels of the intestinal lactase fall during adulthood. In people with lactose intolerance, abdominal pain and bloating occur after ingestion of milk products. Small amounts of butter, yogurt, and cheese may be better tolerated.
- In some people, the disorder is triggered by fatty foods, which can produce intestinal cramping and discomfort.
- Food sensitivities are a common cause. The most common offenders are milk and milk products, grains (wheat and corn), citrus fruits, coffee, and food additives (colorings and flavorings).
- Disruption of colonic microflora and overgrowth of gas-producing bacteria. This may be the result of diets low in fiber, or from use of broad-spectrum antibiotics. Regular consumption of yogurt containing lactobacilli can reduce the number of gas-producing bacteria in the colon and may be beneficial.

Micronutrients

Nutrient	Recommended Daily Dose	Comments
Zinc and magnesium	30 mg zinc, 400 mg magnesium	May reduce cramping and spasms in the colon.
Vitamin B-complex	A balanced supplement containing at least 25 mg thiamin (vitamin B1), riboflavin (vitamin B2), and vitamin B6, as well as 0.4 mg folate	Helps regulate peristalsis and improve function of intestinal smooth muscle.

References

Alun Jones V et al. Food intolerance: a major factor in the pathogenesis of irritable bowel syndrome. *Lancet.* 1982; 2:1115.
Cook IJ et al. Effect of dietary fiber on symptoms and rectosigmoidal motility in patients with irritable bowel syndrome. *Gastroenterol.* 1990; 98:66.
Folwaczny C. Role of zinc in treatment of acute diarrhea. *Z Gastroenterol.* 1996; 34:260.
Gertner D, Powell-Tuck J. Irritable bowel syndrome and food intolerance. *Practitioner.* 1994; 238:499.

Kidney Stones

Diet

In general, the more calcium and oxalate in the urine, the greater the chances of developing kidney stones. Uric acid in the urine can be the 'seed' around which calcium oxalate stones develop. Therefore, people who have a tendency to form kidney stones can reduce the risk by:

- Eating less animal protein. Animal protein increases the amount of calcium, oxalate and uric acid in the urine.
- Increasing the fiber content of the diet, as this can reduce urinary calcium excretion in people who have tendency to form stones. Diets high in fat and salt and low in fiber increase the risk of developing stones.
- Reducing caffeine intake, as high intakes increase calcium excretion into the urine and may promote stone formation. Heavy alcohol use also increases the chance of a kidney stone.
- Drinking plenty of water and other fluids, which increases urinary volume and decreases the concentration of stone-forming substances. People who are susceptible to stones should drink at least 2 L of fluid spread throughout the day.
- Minimizing consumption of foods which are high in oxalate (see Table below).
- Because vitamin C can be metabolized to oxalate, it has been suggested that high intakes of vitamin C might increase the risk of kidney stones. However, oxalate in the urine generally does not increase unless the daily dose of vitamin C is greater than 6 g, and even then only in a small minority of people. In people susceptible to stone formation who are taking high doses of vitamin C, supplemental vitamin B6 and magnesium can reduce the risk of increased oxalate in the urine.

Foods high in oxalates:

- Beans
- Chocolate
- Instant coffee
- Parsley
- Rhubarb
- Spinach
- Carrots

- Celery
- Cucumbers
- Grapefruit
- Peanuts
- Tea

Micronutrients

Nutrient	Recommended Daily Dose	Comments
Vitamin B6	50–100 mg	Required for breakdown of oxalate. In people with high amounts of urinary oxalate, reduces chances of stone formation.
Magnesium	400 mg	Binds with oxalate and decreases the risk of stone formation.

References

Labeeuw M et al. Magnesium in the physiopathology and treatment of renal calcium stones. *Presse Med.* 1987; 16:25.
Mitwalli A et al. Control of hyperoxaluria with large doses of pyridoxine in patients with kidney stones. *Int Urol Nephrol.* 1988: 20:353.
Prien EL, Gershoff SF. Magnesium oxide—pyridoxine therapy for recurrent calcium oxalic calculi. *J Urolog.* 1974; 112:509.
Robertson WG. Diet and calcium stones. *Miner Electrolyte Metab.* 1987; 13:228.

Menopause

Diet

A major concern at the menopause is the loss of bone mineral (mainly calcium) from the skeleton due to the fall in ovarian estrogen secretion. Up to 20% of the bone mineral density can be lost at menopause, which can sharply increase the risk of osteoporosis and bone fractures. Women going through menopause should emphasize rich food sources of calcium, magnesium, and vitamins D and K to maintain the integrity of the skeleton. Also, they should avoid consuming large amounts of phosphorus (found in red meat, processed foods, and cola drinks); too much phosphorus in the diet accelerates mineral loss from the skeleton. Reducing sodium, caffeine, and protein intake can also help maintain body stores of calcium. The loss of estrogen at menopause also causes LDL-cholesterol levels in the blood to rise and levels of HDL-cholesterol to fall, increasing a woman's risk of suffering heart attack and stroke. To keep levels of blood fats in the healthy range, women should reduce the saturated fat content of the diet (by eating less meat, eggs, and whole-fat milk products).

Micronutrients

Nutrient	Recommended Daily Dose	Comments
Vitamin E	400 mg	Can significantly improve hot flashes, fatigue, depression, and vaginal irritation. Vitamin E in creams can be used topically in the vagina to reduce itching and irritation
Gamma-linolenic acid (GLA)	As 2–4 g evening primrose oil (EPO)	Can be effective in reducing hot flashes, vaginal irritation, and mood swings.
Calcium and vitamin D	800–1000 mg calcium; 10 μg vitamin D	Reduces loss of mineral content of the bones and helps maintain bone integrity.

References

Chapuy MC et al. Vitamin D_3 and calcium to prevent hip fractures in elderly women. *N Engl J Med.* 1992; 327:1637.
Dawson-Hughes B. Calcium supplementation and bone loss: a review of the controlled clinical trials. *Am J Clin Nutr.* 1991; 54:274.
Finkler RS. The effect of vitamin E in the menopause. *J Clin Endocrinol Metab.* 1949; 9:89.
Wenger NK et al. Cardiovascular health and disease in women. *N Engl Med J.* 1993; 329:247

Migraine

Diet

Foods often trigger migraine. People with migraine should try to identify potential food sensitivities; elimination diets can pinpoint the offending foods (p. 146). Reactive hypoglycemia may also trigger migraines (p. 166).

Substances that Commonly Trigger Migraine	Food Sources
Vasoactive amines are substances that cause blood vessel dilation (tyramine and phenylethylamine are commonest forms)	Red wine, aged cheese, chicken liver, pickled herring, sausage, processed meat, sour cream, chocolate, bananas, pork, onions
Lactose (milk sugar) can cause migraines in people who are lactose intolerant	Dairy products
Ethanol	Alcoholic beverages
Aspartame	Artificially sweetened products
Nitrites (meat preservatives and colorings)	Sausage, salami, processed meats
Caffeine	Coffee, soft drinks, chocolate, tea
Copper (foods with high copper content can dilate blood vessels and stimulate migraine)	Chocolate, nuts, shellfish, wheat germ
Monosodium glutamate (flavor enhancer)	Processed foods

Micronutrients

Nutrient	Recommended Daily Dose	Comments
Magnesium and vitamin B6	400–600 mg magnesium; 50 mg vitamin B6	Low levels of magnesium in the body may increase the risk of blood vessel constriction and spasm. Particularly effective in women who have migraines associated with the menstrual period or during pregnancy.
Omega-3 fatty acids	2–4 g EPA (as fish oil capsules)	May reduce frequency and intensity of migraines.
Vitamin D and calcium	10 μg vitamin D; 600 mg calcium	May reduce frequency and intensity of migraines.

References

Dexter JD et al. The five hour glucose tolerance test and effect of low sucrose diet in migraine. *Headache.* 1978; 18:91.
Glueck CJ et al. Amelioration of severe migraine with omega-3 fatty acids: A double-blind, placebo-controlled clinical trial. *Am J Clin Nutr.* 1986; 43:710.
Peikert A et al. Prophylaxis of migraine with oral magnesium: results from a prospective, multi-center, placebo-controlled and double-blind randomized study. *Cephalalgia.* 1996; 16:257.
Taubert K. Magnesium in migraine. Results of a multicenter pilot study. *Fortschr Med.* 1994; 112:328.
Thys-Jacobs S. Alleviation of migraines with therapeutic vitamin D and calcium. *Headache.* 1994; 34:590.
Vaughan TR. The role of food in the pathogenesis of migraine headache. *Clin Rev Allergy.* 1994; 12:167.

Multiple Sclerosis

Diet

In people with multiple sclerosis (MS), particularly at the beginning of the disease, a low-fat diet (< 15 g fat/day) may slow progression and reduce the severity of symptoms. Along with reducing total fat intake, polyunsaturated fats (cold-pressed nut and seed oils) should be substituted for saturated fats. Because oxidative damage from free radicals may play a role in MS, diets should be high in natural antioxidants (such as vitamin E, C, carotenoids, and selenium). Food sensitivities may ag gravate MS (common offending foods are milk and chocolate), and an elimination diet (p. 146) with identification and avoidance of offending foods may be beneficial.

Micronutrients

Nutrient	Recommended Daily Dose	Comments
Vitamin E and selenium	400–1200 mg vitamin E; 200 μg selenium	Antioxidants may protect against myelin degeneration.
Omega-3 fatty acids	1–2 g EPA (as fish oil capsules)	May slow progression and reduce severity.
Vitamin B-complex	Balanced formula containing 50 mg vitamin B6, 50 mg thiamin (vitamin B1), and 0.4 mg folic acid	Deficiencies of vitamin B6, niacin (vitamin B3), and folic acid can aggravate symptoms.
Vitamin B12	1 mg/week via intramuscular injection	Vitamin B12 is essential for production of fatty acids that make up myelin. Deficiency can aggravate MS.
Gamma-linolenic acid (GLA)	1–3 g evening primrose oil (EPO)	Supplementation may be beneficial, particularly as part of a diet low in saturated fat.

References

Cendrowski W. Multiple sclerosis and MaxEPA. *Br J Clin Prac.* 1986; 40:365.
Mai J et al. High dose antioxidant supplementation to multiple sclerosis patients. *Biol Trace Element Res.* 1990; 24:109.
Ransohoff RM et al. Vitamin B12 deficiency and multiple sclerosis. *Lancet.* 1990; 335:1285.
Swank RL, Dugan BB. Effect of low saturated fat diet in early and late cases of multiple sclerosis. *Lancet.* 1990; 336:37.

Muscle Cramps

Diet

Diets in the industrialized countries are often low in magnesium, calcium, and potassium, and many commonly-used drugs, including diuretics and laxatives, increase losses of these important minerals. Low levels of potassium, magnesium, and/or calcium in muscles can trigger spasm and cramps. Daily consumption of fruits, vegetables, low-fat milk products, and whole grains will provide generous amounts of these minerals. Adequate intake of fluid during hot weather and exercise will eliminate cramping due to dehydration.

Micronutrients

Nutrient	Recommended Daily Dose	Comments
Vitamin E	200–400 mg	Reduces nighttime leg cramps. Also helps reduce muscle cramps during pregnancy. During strenuous exercise, oxidative stress contributes to muscle fatigue and cramps; vitamin E helps protect against oxidative stress.
Calcium/ magnesium	1000 mg/400 mg	Low levels of calcium increase irritability of nerves and muscles and can produce muscle cramps. Particularly effective for pregnancy-associated leg cramps when given with magnesium.
Vitamin B-complex	Balanced supplement containing 25–50 mg thiamin (vitamin B1), niacin (vitamin B3), and pantothenic acid	Supports optimal energy metabolism in muscles and helps clear by-products of exercise (such as lactate) that cause muscles to cramp.

References

Hammar M et al. Calcium treatment of leg cramps in pregnancy. Effect on clinical symptoms and total serum and ionized serum calcium concentrations. *Acta Obstet Gynecol Scand*. 1981; 60:345.

Cathcart RF. Leg cramps and vitamin E. *JAMA*. 1972; 219:216.

Obesity

Diet

Diets high in fat increase the risk of weight gain. While protein and carbohydrate each contain 4 kcal/g, fat has more than double that amount—9 kcal/g. Moreover, dietary fat is efficiently stored as body fat, while protein and carbohydrate must first be converted to fat before storage, a process that requires energy and is less efficient. In order for the average person to lose about 0.5 kg of body fat per week, energy intake must be cut by about 500 kcal per day. Reducing caloric intake to between 1000–1500 kcal/day, particularly when combined with moderate exercise, produces a gradual but steady loss of body fat and weight. Fiber adds nondigestible bulk, so that eating fiber-rich foods results in satiety with lower caloric intake, encouraging weight loss. Fruits, vegetables, whole grains, and legumes are fiber-rich foods that should be a large part of diets for weight loss. Alcoholic drinks contain large amounts of calories; for example, a medium-sized glass of dry wine contains about 120 kcal. The following plan provides a healthy way to trim body fat and will usually produce a weight loss of about 0.5–1 kg of body fat per week:

- Diet should be:
  - low-fat (less than 20 g fat/day) and low-calorie (about 1000 cal/day);
  - one third of calories should be from high-quality protein (low-fat milk products, eggs, fish);
  - one half of calories from carbohydrates (whole grains, fruits, vegetables, peas, and beans);
- Combine with 30–45 minutes of aerobic exercise (walking, jogging, swimming) at least three to four times per week.

Micronutrients

Nutrient	Recommended Daily Dose	Comments
Fiber (such as guar gum)	1–2 g with each meal	Increases feeling of satiety and may help reduce caloric intake. Take with ample fluids.
Multivitamin/mineral supplement	Complete, balanced formula including 100–200 mg vitamin C	Ensures micronutrient balance during hypocaloric dieting.

References

Krotkiewski M. Effect of guar gum on body-weight, hunger ratings and metabolism in obese subjects. *Br J Nutr.* 1984; 52:97.

Naylor GJ et al. A double blind placebo controlled trial of ascorbic acid in obesity. *Nutr Health.* 1985; 4:25.

Pi-Sunyer FX. Medical hazards of obesity. *Ann Intern Med.* 1993; 119:655.

Rigaud D et al. Overweight treated with energy restriction and a dietary fibre supplement: A 6-month randomized, double-blind, placebo-controlled trial. *Int J Obes.* 1990; 14:763.

Rosenbaum M et al. Obesity. *N Engl J Med.* 1997; 337:396.

Oral Aphthae

Diet

In certain individuals, aphthae may be caused by food sensitivity. An elimination diet can identify the offending foods, which can then be avoided. Highly acidic foods (e.g., tomatoes, citrus fruits) can produce aphthae in susceptible people. Stress can also be a trigger. Because they compete with and reduce the number of oral streptococci, *Lactobacilli* in yogurt and other fermented milk products can reduce frequency and severity of aphthae.

Micronutrients

Nutrient	Recommended Daily Dose	Comments
Zinc	30–60 mg	Can help prevent aphthae, particularly in people who have marginal zinc status.
Vitamin B-complex	Balanced supplement containing all the B vitamins; ample folic acid and vitamin B12 are particularly important	B vitamins promote health and strength of the oral mucosa.
Vitamin A	2000 μg	Helps to maintain the health and integrity of oral tissues.

References

Endre L. Successful treatment of recurrent ulcerative stomatitis, associated with cellular immune defect and hypozincaemia, by oral administration of zinc sulfate *Orv Hetil.* 1990; 131:475.

Wang SW et al. The trace element zinc and aphthosis. The determination of plasma zinc and the treatment of aphthosis with zinc. *Rev Stomatol Chir Maxillofac.* 1986; 87:339.

Wray D. Aphthous stomatitis is linked to mechanical injuries, iron and vitamin deficiencies and certain HLA types. *JAMA.* 1982; 247:774.

Wray D, Ferguson MM, Mason DK, Hutcheon AW, Dagg JH. Recurrent aphthae; treatment with vitamin B12, folic acid and iron. *BMJ.* 1975; 5:490.

Wray D, Vlagopoulos TP, Siraganian RP. Food allergens and basophil histamine release in recurrent aphthous stomatitis. *Oral Surg Oral Med Oral Path.* 1982; 54:388.

Oral Contraceptives

Diet

Oral contraceptive pills (OCPs) may contribute to hyperlipidemia and impaired glucose tolerance. Women using OCPs need to be particularly careful to minimize consumption of saturated and hydrogenated fats, as well as refined carbohydrates and sugar, to help maintain control of blood lipids and glucose.
In addition, OCPs have wide-ranging effects on micronutrient status.

There is an increased requirement for:	
Thiamin (vitamin B1), riboflavin (vitamin B2), and vitamin B12	Interferes with metabolism and increases requirements for these B vitamins.
Vitamin B6	Interferes with metabolism. Needs for vitamin B6 are two to ten times higher than in women taking OCPs compared to women not taking them.
Folic acid	Interferes with metabolism and increases requirements. Women taking OCPs are often deficient in folate. Folate deficiency is particularly dangerous to the developing baby during early pregnancy, and can cause birth defects (see p. 88). Women should wait 3–6 months after stopping OCPs before attempting pregnancy, and during these months a vitamin B-complex with 0.8 mg folic acid should be taken to replenish body stores.
Vitamin C	May lower tissue and blood levels.
Zinc and magnesium	May interfere with metabolism and increase requirements for these minerals. Many women taking OCPs are deficient in zinc and magnesium.

There may be lower requirement for:	
Vitamin A	Increases levels of the vitamin A transport protein and vitamin A in the blood. Women taking OCPs should avoid high doses of vitamin A, because OCPs can potentially increase the chances of toxicity from vitamin A.
Vitamin K	Increases levels of the vitamin K–dependent clotting proteins in the blood, increasing the risk of blood clots.
Copper	Increases circulating copper levels in the blood.

Micronutrients

Nutrient	Recommended Daily Dose
Vitamin B-complex	Complete formula containing at least 5 mg thiamin (vitamin B1) and riboflavin (vitamin B2), 25 mg vitamin B6, 0.4 mg folate, and 10 µg vitamin B12
Vitamin C	100–250 mg
Multimineral supplement	Should contain at least 250 mg magnesium and 15 mg zinc.

References

Leklem JE. Vitamin B6 requirement and oral contraceptive use-a concern? *J Nutr.* 1986; 116:475.

Prasad AS et al. Effect of oral contraceptives on nutrients: vitamin B6, B12 and folic acid. *Am J Obstet Gynaecol.* 1976; 125:1063.

Thorp VJ. Effect of oral contraceptive agents on vitamin and mineral requirements. *J Am Diet Assoc.* 1980; 76:581.

Osteoarthritis

Diet

Aspirin and other popular nonsteroidal anti-inflammatory drugs used by people with joint aches disrupt the integrity of the gastrointestinal mucosa and may increase the ability of food allergens to cross into the bloodstream. This may increase the risk of food sensitivities that can worsen arthritis. The most commonly implicated foods are in the nightshade family—potato, tomato, eggplant, and peppers. Being overweight places a greater load on joints and can contribute to osteoarthritis in the hips, back, and knees. Fruits and vegetables are good sources of vitamins C and E; high intake of these antioxidant nutrients is associated with lower risk of osteoarthritis. Maintaining ample body stores of vitamin D (dietary intake + sunlight exposure) can also reduce risk.

Micronutrients

Nutrient	Recommended Daily Dose	Comments
Vitamin E	400–800 mg	Can help reduce pain and stiffness and improve joint mobility. May slow progression of osteoarthritis.
Vitamin D	5–10 μg	May slow progression of osteoarthritis.
Multimineral supplement	Balanced formula containing generous amounts of calcium, magnesium, and 100–200 μg selenium	Supports repair of the articular cartilage and underlying bone.
Vitamin B-complex	Complete formula containing at least 0.8 mg folic acid and 25 μg vitamin B12	May help provide relief of symptoms.

References

Flynn MA The effect of folate and cobalamin on osteoarthritic hands. *J Am Coll Nutr.* 1994; 13:351.
Jameson S et al. Pain relief and selenium balance in patients with connective tissue disease and osteoarthrosis: A double-blind selenium tocopherol supplementation study. *Nutr Res.* 1985(Suppl 1):391.
Machtey I, Ouaknine L. Tocopherol in osteoarthritis: a controlled pilot study. *J Am Geriat Soc.* 1978; 26:328.
McAlindon TE et al. Do antioxidant nutrients protect against development and progression of knee osteoarthritis? *Arthritis Rheum.* 1996; 39:648.
McAlindon TE et al. Relation of dietary intake and serum levels of vitamin D to progression of osteoarthritis of the knee among participants of the Framingham study. *Ann Intern Med.* 1996; 125:353.

Osteoporosis

Diet

Although osteoporotic fractures occur in the elderly, prevention begins early in life. Achieving peak bone mass during childhood and early adulthood ensures that reserves of bone mineral will be available for later years. Foods rich in the nutrients needed to build bone—particularly calcium, magnesium, manganese, and vitamins A and D—should be consumed regularly during childhood and adolescence. During adulthood, low-fat milk products enriched with vitamin D should be consumed daily to provide calcium and minerals. Even in women who are taking postmenopausal estrogen replacement, additional calcium will help maintain bone density. Diets in the industrialized countries contain large amounts of several food components that increase calcium losses and may increase the risk of osteoporosis. Phosphorus (in meats, processed foods, soft drinks) can interfere with bone remodeling and increase losses of calcium. Similarly, high intakes of protein, sodium, caffeine, and alcohol increase losses of body calcium. Together with widespread dietary deficiencies of vitamin D, calcium, and minerals, these dietary patterns are responsible for the epidemic of osteoporosis among older individuals in the industrialized countries.

Micronutrients

Nutrient	Recommended Daily Dose	Comments
Calcium	1 g; 1.5 g for postmenopausal women	Supplemental calcium should be taken in divided doses during the day, with about half of the total dose taken at bedtime.
Vitamin D	10–20 µg	Increases absorption of calcium. Regular exposure to sunshine helps maintain vitamin D levels. Supplements are especially valuable in dark, winter months or for housebound people.
Magnesium	300–500 mg	Activates enzymes essential in bone formation. Magnesium deficiency is common in osteoporosis.

Nutrient	Recommended Daily Dose	Comments
Multimineral preparation	Should contain ample amounts of manganese, zinc, and copper	The trace minerals manganese, copper, and zinc are important in bone maintenance.

References

Chapuy MC et al. Vitamin D3 and calcium to prevent hip fractures in elderly women. *N Engl J Med.* 1992; 327:1637.

Dawson-Hughes B et al. Effect of vitamin D supplementation on wintertime and overall bone loss in healthy postmenopausal women. *Ann Int Med.* 1991; 115:505.

King J. Does poor zinc nutriture retard skeletal growth and mineralization in adolescents? *Am J Clin Nutr.* 1996; 64:375.

Münzenberg KJ, Koch W. Mineralogic aspects in the treatment of osteoporosis with magnesium. *J Am Coll Nutr.* 1989; 8:461.

Nieves JW et al. Calcium potentiates the effect of estrogen and calcitonin on bone mass: review and analysis. *Am J Clin Nutr.* 1997; 67:18.

Teegarden D, Weaver CM. Calcium supplementation increases bone density in adolescent girls. *Nutr Rev.* 1994; 52:171.

Villareal DT et al. Subclinical vitamin D deficiency in postmenopausal women with low vertebral bone mass. *J Clin Endocrinol Metab.* 1991; 72:628.

Otitis Media

Diet

In infants and children with frequent middle ear infections, food or environmental allergies should be investigated. Allergy to cow's milk can cause swelling of the nasopharynx mucosa and eustachian tube which may increase risk of infection. Eliminating the offending food can prevent reinfection. Optimal nutrition can support the immune system and reduce the chances of recurrent infections and the need for antibiotics.

Micronutrients*

Nutrient	Recommended Daily Dose	Comments
Multivitamin/mineral supplement for children	Should contain 400 μg vitamin A and 10 mg vitamin E; 10 mg zinc and 10 mg iron	Maintains optimal functioning of the immune system.
Vitamin C	250 mg	Supports the immune system and helps fight infection.

* To reduce or prevent inner ear infections in children aged 1–6 years; older children and adults may need higher doses

References

Dallman PR. Iron deficiency and the immune response. *Am J Clin Nutr.* 1987; 46:329.

Grimble RF. Effect of antioxidative vitamins on immune function with clinical applications. *Int J Vitam Nutr Res.* 1997; 67:312.

Jeng KCG et al. Supplementation with vitamins C and E enhances cytokine production by peripheral blood mononuclear cells in healthy adults. *Am J Clin Nutr.*1996; 64:960.

Solomons NW. Mild zinc deficiency produces an imbalance between cell-mediated and humoral immunity. *Nutr Rev.* 1998: 56:27.

Parkinson's Disease

Diet

A low protein diet can be beneficial in Parkinson's disease. L-dopa is one of several amino acids that compete for uptake into the brain from the bloodstream. During L-dopa therapy, restricting dietary protein reduces competition from other amino acids and allows more L-dopa to enter the brain. One limitation of L-dopa therapy is that its beneficial effects may unpredictably wax and wane through the day—protein restriction can reduce these daily fluctuations and make L-dopa therapy more effective, particularly if most of the daily protein is eaten in the evening meal. High doses of vitamin B6 may decrease the effectiveness of L-dopa therapy and should generally be avoided. Oxidation from free radicals appears to play a role in Parkinson's disease. Diets high in natural antioxidants (such as vitamins E and C and the carotenoids) may reduce the risk of developing Parkinson's disease, and, in people with the disease, may slow progression.

Micronutrients

Nutrient	Recommended Daily Dose	Comments
Vitamin E and selenium	800–2400 mg vitamin E; 200–400 μg selenium	Antioxidants may protect against nerve cell degeneration. Begin with 400 IU and gradually increase over several weeks.
Vitamin C	1–4 g	May improve symptoms, especially alongside treatment with L-dopa.
Vitamin B-complex	Balanced formula containing 0.4 mg folic acid, 50 mg niacin (vitamin B3)	Deficiencies of niacin (vitamin B3) and folic acid often develop in people with Parkinson's disease, and low body stores of these B vitamins can worsen symptoms.
Gamma-linolenic acid (GLA)	As evening primrose oil (EPO), 2–4 g/day	May be effective in reducing trembling.
L-Methionine	1–5 g	Start with 1 g/day and increase dose over several weeks. Can increase ease of movement, strength, mood, and sleep.

References

Fahn S. An open trial of high-dosage antioxidants in early Parkinson's disease. *Am J Clin Nutr.* 1991; 53:380.
Grimes JD et al. Prevention of progression of Parkinson's disease with antioxidative therapy. *Prog Neuropsychopharmacol Biol Psychiatry*. 1988; 12:165.
Kempster PA, Wahlqvist ML. Dietary factors in the management of Parkinson's disease. *Nutr Rev*. 1994; 52:51.
Smythies JR, Halsey JH. Treatment of Parkinson's disease with L-methionine. *South Med J*. 1984; 77:1577.

Peptic Ulcer

Diet

Dietary factors play a central role in ulcer frequency and severity. High intakes of sugar and refined carbohydrate can contribute to ulcers. Milk, traditionally recommended to reduce acidity, actually produces only a transient rise in pH which is often followed by a large rebound increase in acid secretion, which can worsen ulcers. Heavy alcohol consumption can cause erosions and ulceration of the stomach lining. Both decaffeinated and regular coffee can aggravate heartburn and ulcers in many people. Food sensitivities (such as allergy to cow's milk) may contribute to ulcer formation; identifying and avoiding the offending foods often improves healing and may prevent recurrence. Raw cabbage juice contains large amounts of S-methylmethionine and glutamine, two amino acids that can speed healing of ulcers. Drinking 0.5 L of raw cabbage juice a day may help promote healing. In cases of ulcer due to *Helicobacter pylori*, optimal nutrition can maintain the health of the protec tive lining of the stomach and duodenum. It can also support the immune system to increase resistance to chronic *Helicobacter* infection.

Micronutrients

Nutrient	Recommended Daily Dose	Comments
Vitamin A	8000–10 000 μg	Supports the gastric mucosa, may protect against ulceration and promote healing. High doses of vitamin A should only be taken under the advice of a physician.
Vitamin E	400 mg	Helps protect against ulcer development and may aid healing of ulcers both in the stomach and duodenum.
Zinc	30–60 mg	Speeds healing of ulcers.
L-Glutamine	1–1.5 g	Glutamine promotes healing of the gastric and duodenal mucosa.

References

Aldoori WH et al. Prospective study of diet and the risk of duodenal ulcer in men. *Am J Epidemiol.* 1997; 145:42.

Escolar G. Zinc compounds, a new treatment in peptic ulcer. *Drugs Exp Clin Res.* 1989; 15:83.

Kaess H et al. Food intolerance in duodenal ulcer patients, nonulcer dyspeptic patients and healthy subjects. A prospective study. *Klin Wochenschr.* 1988; 66:208.

Katschinski BD et al. Duodenal ulcer and refined carbohydrate intake: a case-control study assessing dietary fibre and refined sugar intake. *Gut.* 1990; 31:993.

Moutairy AR, Tariq M. Effect of vitamin E and selenium on hypothermic restraint stress and chemically-induced ulcers. *Dig Dis Sci.* 1996; 41:1165.

Patty I et al. Controlled trial of vitamin A therapy in gastric ulcer. *Lancet.* 1982; 2:876.

Tovey F. Diet and duodenal ulcer. *J Gastroenterol Hepatol.* 1994; 9:177.

Peripheral Vascular Disease

Diet

Follow the diet recommendations for atherosclerosis (p. 127 ff.). In general, saturated fat in the diet should be replaced with cold-pressed plant and seed oils which provide essential fatty acids and can aid circulation. Eating fish two to three times per week provides omega-3 fatty acids that aid in maintaining blood circulation. Refined carbohydrates should be replaced with complex carbohydrates from vegetables and whole grains, to provide additional fiber.

Micronutrients

Nutrient	Recommended Daily Dose	Comments
Vitamin E	400 mg	Decreases tendency for platelet aggregation and improves circulation. May reduce calf pain and cramping in people with peripheral vascular disease.
Niacin (vitamin B3) (in form of nicotinic acid)	100–200 mg	Lowers LDL-cholesterol in the blood and raises HDL-cholesterol, thereby reducing atherogenic risk. Produces peripheral vasodilation that aids circulation. Take with meals.
Vitamin B-complex	Balanced formula containing 0.4–0.8 mg folic acid	Reduces plasma homocysteine and may improve circulation.
Omega-3 fatty acids	2–3 g of EPA and DHA (as fish oil capsules)	Decreases platelet aggregation and risk of thrombosis; improves circulation.

References

Jandak J, Steiner M, Richardson PD. Alpha tocopherol, an effective inhibitor of platelet adhesion. *Blood.* 1989; 73:141.

Luria MH. Effect of low-dose niacin on high density lipoprotein cholesterol and total cholesterol/high density lipoprotein cholesterol concentration. *Arch Intern Med.* 1988; 148:2493.

Peterson JC, Spence JD. Vitamins and progression of atherosclerosis in hyperhomocysteinemia. *Lancet.* 1998; 351:263.

Premenstrual Syndrome

Diet

Many women with Premenstrual Syndrome (PMS) experience cravings for refined carbohydrates and sugar. Carbohydrates may improve mood by enhancing production of the neurotransmitter serotonin in the brain. However, eating large amounts of sugar and refined carbohydrate can increase water retention and weight gain. By increasing intake of tryptophan-rich foods (the amino acid tryptophan is converted to serotonin in the brain), women with PMS can reduce cravings for carbohydrate, and may avoid these problems. Heavy alcohol and caffeine intake during the two weeks leading up to menstruation can aggravate the headache and irritability associated with PMS. A diet low in salt may reduce fluid retention. High intakes of magnesium may help reduce the symptoms of PMS: rich sources are seeds, nuts, whole grains, and vegetables. Iron deficiency is especially likely in women who have heavy bleeding during their periods. Women with heavy periods should consume rich dietary sources of iron (lean meats, liver, dark-green leafy vegetables) to replace losses of iron in menstrual bleeding.

Micronutrients

Nutrient	Recommended Daily Dose	Comments
Gamma-linolenic acid (GLA)	As 2–4 g evening primrose oil (EPO)	May reduce severity of symptoms.
Vitamin B6 and magnesium	50–100 mg vitamin B6, 400 mg magnesium	Marginal deficiency can aggravate symptoms. Supplements can reduce nervous tension, breast pain, and weight gain. Helps reduce severity of menstrual cramps.
Omega-3 fatty acids	EPA as 1–3 g fish oil	May help reduce painful menstrual cramping.
Vitamin C with bioflavonoids	100–250 mg vitamin C with a bioflavonoid complex	May help reduce heavy bleeding during menstrual periods.
Vitamin E	400 mg	May help reduce severity of breast tenderness and menstrual cramps.

References

Budeiri D et al. Is evening primrose oil of value in the treatment of premenstrual syndrome? *Control Clin Trials.* 1996; 17:60.

Cohen JD, Ruben HW. Functional menorrhagia: treatment with bioflavonoids and vitamin C. *Curr Ther Res.* 1960; 2:539.

Deutch B. Menstrual pain in Danish women correlated with low n-3 polyunsaturated fatty acid intake. *Eur J Clin Nutr.* 1995; 49:508.

Doll H. Vitamin B6 and the premenstrual syndrome: a randomized cross-over trial. *J R Coll Gen Pract.* 1989; 39:364.

Facchinetti F et al. Oral magnesium successfully relieves premenstrual mood changes. *Obstet Gynecol.* 1992; 78: 177.

Fontana-Klaiber H, Hogg B. Therapeutic effects of magnesium in dysmenorrhea. *Schweiz Rundsch Med Prax.* 1990; 79:491.

Harel Z et al. Supplementation with omega-3 polyunsaturated fatty acids in the management of dysmenorrhea in adolescents. *Am J Obstet Gynecol.* 1996; 174:1335.

Kendall KE, Schnurr PP. The effects of vitamin B6 supplementation of premenstrual symptoms. *Obstet Gynecol.* 1987; 70:145.

London RS. Efficacy of alpha-tocopherol in the treatment of the premenstrual syndrome. *J Reprod Med.* 1987; 32:400.

Prostatic Hypertrophy

Diet

High-fat diets, particularly saturated fat from animal sources (meat, eggs, dairy products), promotes enlargement of the prostate, and may also increase the risk of developing prostate cancer. Diets high in fruits and vegetables, particularly those rich in lycopene (a carotenoid found in large amounts in tomatoes) reduce the risk of prostate enlargement and cancer. Overactivity of prostaglandins within the prostate gland may contribute to enlargement. Substituting high quality, cold-pressed plant oils for saturated fat in the diet, along with eating fresh fish two to three times per week, will provide important essential polyunsaturated fatty acids (PUFAs). The essential fatty acids and their metabolites—GLA, EPA and DHA—can decrease the activity of these prostaglandins (see p. 79), and may reduce enlargement and improve symptoms.

Micronutrients

Nutrient	Recommended Daily Dose	Comments
Vitamin E	200–400 mg	Supplementation may reduce risk of enlargement and prostate cancer.
Zinc	30–60 mg	Impaired zinc metabolism within the prostate gland may contribute to enlargement. Supplementation may reduce gland size and improve symptoms.
Essential fatty acids (EFAs)	GLA as 2–4 g evening primrose oil (EPO); 1–3 g EPA and DHA as fish oil capsules	May reduce gland size and improve symptoms.
Amino acids	Combination of three amino acids: L-glycine, L-alanine, and L-glutamic acid; each taken at a dose of 500 mg/day	May reduce size of the gland and improve symptoms

References

Dumrau F. Benign prostatic hyperplasia: Amino acid therapy for symptomatic relief. *Am J Geriatr.* 1962; 10:426.
Fahim MS et al. Zinc treatment for the reduction of hyperplasia of the prostate. *Fed Proc.* 1976; 35:361.
Giles G, Ireland P. Diet, nutrition and prostate cancer. *Int J Cancer.* 1997; 10:13.
Giovanucci E, Rimm EB, Colditz GA et al. A prospective study of dietary fat and risk of prostate cancer. *JNCI.* 1993; 85:1571.
Heinonen OP et al. Prostate cancer and supplementation with alpha-tocopherol and beta-carotene. *J Natl Cancer Inst* 1998; 90:440–446.

Psoriasis

Diet

In the skin of people with psoriasis, metabolism of essential fatty acids (EFAs) is abnormal. Production of EPA and DHA, the omega-3 fatty acids derived from dietary linolenic acid (p. 79) is impaired. Therefore, regular consumption of fish rich in EPA and DHA may be beneficial. The diet should also be low in saturated fat and hydrogenated fat. Vegetarian diets can dramatically improve psoriasis in some people; these diets tend to be low in protein (protein can aggravate the condition) and high in EFAs. Because food sensitivities may promote psoriasis, food sensitivities should be determined—some people improve on careful food-elimination diets. Alcohol can aggravate psoriasis in certain individuals.

Micronutrients

Nutrient	Recommended Daily Dose	Comments
Omega-3 fatty acids	As fish oil capsules, 1–1.5 g EPA and DHA	Can reduce proliferation and inflammation. Skin salves containing EPA can also be applied to patches. Take with at least 100 IU vitamin E.
Selenium and zinc	200 µg selenium, 50 mg zinc	People with psoriasis often have low blood levels of selenium. Zinc and selenium supplements can reduce skin inflammation, itching, and redness. These nutrients can also be effective when used topically as selenium sulfide or zinc oxide salves.
Vitamins A and D	8000 µg vitamin A and 20 µg of vitamin D	Vitamins A and D play central roles in the regulation and control of skin cell growth, and supplementation can help clear psoriasis. Calcitriol, the active form of vitamin D3, is effective in both oral and topical treatments. Skin salves containing vitamins A and D can be applied directly to psoriatic plaques. High doses of vitamin A should only be taken under the advice of a physician.

References

Bittiner SB et al. A double-blind, randomised, placebo-controlled trial of fish oil in psoriasis. *Lancet.* 1988; 1:378.

Lowe KE. Vitamin D and psoriasis. *Nutr Rev.* 1992; 50:138.

Majewski S et al. Decreased levels of vitamin A in serum of patients with psoriasis. *Arch Dermatol Res.* 1989; 280:499.

Naldi L. Dietary factors and the risk of psoriasis. *Br J Dermatol.* 1996; 134:101.

Stewart DG, Lewis HM. Vitamin D analogues and psoriasis. *J Clin Pharm Ther.* 1996; 21:143.

Rheumatoid Arthritis

Diet

Food sensitivities are a common cause of rheumatoid arthritis (RA). People with RA should determine if food sensitivities are present by means of an elimination diet (p. 146 ff.). Identification and avoidance of offending foods can produce dramatic improvements in symptoms and function. Aspirin and other nonsteroidal anti-inflammatory drugs damage the gastrointestinal mucosa and increase the ability of allergens to cross into the bloodstream, and thereby may aggravate food sensitivities that often contribute to RA. Diets high in essential polyunsaturated fats and low in saturated fat can increase tissue production of anti-inflammatory prostaglandins and leukotrienes that reduce pain and swelling. Cold-water fish should be eaten two to three times per week to provide omega-3-fatty acids to reduce inflammation. For some people with RA, a semivegetarian diet (including fish, but no meat, milk, or eggs) can significantly reduce inflammation and halt progression of RA. In advanced cases of RA, because nutrient absorption from the gut is impaired (due to the autoimmune reaction in the intestine), nutrient deficiencies—particularly of the B vitamins and trace minerals—are common.

Micronutrients

Nutrient	Recommended Daily Dose	Comments
Omega-3 fatty acids	2–3 g EPA (as fish oil capsules)	Reduces inflammation and may lessen stiffness and pain. Supports healing of the damaged synovium.
Vitamin E	400–800 mg	Protects against oxidative damage, reduces inflammation, and may provide effective pain relief.
Vitamin C	1–2 g	Protects against oxidative damage and helps regulate disordered immune function. May stimulate repair of damaged cartilage and speed healing.

Micronutrients

Nutrient	Recommended Daily Dose	Comments
Pantothenic acid	0.5–2 g (as calcium pantothenate)	Begin with 0.5 g/day and increase gradually until improvement is noted. Can reduce pain, stiffness, and disability.
L-Histidine	0.5–1.5 g	May help reduce joint pain and stiffness.
Multimineral formula	High-dose formula with 2–6 mg copper, 15–30 mg zinc, 100–200 μg selenium	Copper stimulates the enzyme superoxide dismutase (SOD), which can reduce oxidative damage, stiffness, and pain. Zinc and selenium may reduce inflammation and help relieve symptoms.

References

Belch JJF et al. Effects of altering dietary essential fatty acids on requirements for non-steroidal anti-inflammatory drugs in patients with rheumatoid arthritis: A double-blind placebo controlled study. *Annals of the Rheumatic Diseases*. 1988; 47:96.

Darlington LG, Ramsey NW. Review of dietary therapy for rheumatoid arthritis. *Compr Ther.* 1994; 20:490.

General Practitioner's Research Group. Calcium pantothenate in arthritis conditions. *Practitioner.* 1980; 224:208.

Honkanen VEA et al. Plasma zinc and copper concentrations in rheumatoid arthritis: influence of dietary factors and disease activity. *Am J Clin Nutr.* 1991; 54:1082.

Kjeldsen Kragh J et al. Vegetarian diet for patients with rheumatoid arthritis- status: two years after introduction of the diet. *Clin Rheumatol.* 1994; 13:475.

Kolarz GO et al. High dose vitamin E in chronic polyarthritis. *Akt Rheumatol.* 1990; 15:233.

Kremer JM, Bigaouette J. Nutrient intake of patients with rheumatoid arthritis is deficient in pyridoxine, zinc, copper, and magnesium. *J Rheumatol.* 1996; 23:990.

Morgan SL. Supplementation with folic acid during methotrexate therapy for rheumatoid arthritis. A double blind, placebo-controlled trial. *Ann Intern Med.* 1994; 121:833.

Peretz A et al. Effects of zinc supplementation on the phagocytic functions of polymorphonuclears in patients with inflammatory rheumatic diseases. *J Trace Elem Electrolytes Health Dis.* 1994; 8:189.

Pinals RS et al. Treatment of rheumatoid arthritis with L-histidine: A randomized, placebo-controlled, double-blind trial. *J Rheumatol.* 1977; 4:414.

Simkin PA. Treatment of rheumatoid arthritis with oral zinc sulphate. *Agents Action.* 1981(Suppl 8):587.

Sperling RI. Eicosanoids in rheumatoid arthritis. *Rheum Dis Clin North Am.* 1995; 21:741.

Tarp U. Selenium in rheumatoid arthritis. A review. *Analyst.* 1995; 120:877.

Appendix

Drug–Micronutrient Interactions

Drug	Micronutrient	Interaction
Angiotension-converting-enzyme inhibitors	Potassium	Increases blood potassium level
Adrenocorticotropin hormone	Potassium	Increases urinary potassium excretion
	Vitamin B6	Increases urinary B6 excretion
Adriamycin	Coenzyme Q10	Increases CoQ10 requirements
Alcohol	B-Complex and fat-soluble vitamins	Reduces vitamin absorption impairs metabolism
	Magnesium	Increases urinary magnesium excretion
	Zinc	Reduces zinc absorption and increases urinary excretion
Allopurinol	Iron	Enhances storage of liver iron
Aminoglycosides	Potassium, Magnesium, Calcium, Zinc	Increases urinary mineral excretion
	Vitamin K, Biotin	Reduces endogenous vitamin production by colonic bacteria
Aminopterin	Folate	Impairs vitamin metabolism
Amitryptilline	Riboflavin	Impairs vitamin metabolism
Amphotericin B	Potassium, Magnesium	Increases urinary mineral excretion
Androgens	Calcium	Reduces urinary calcium excretion, may produce hypercalcemia

Drug	Micronutrient	Interaction
Antacids	Vitamin B-complex, Choline, Vitamin A, Vitamin C, Calcium, Phosphorus, Iron, Zinc, Flouride	Reduces vitamin and mineral absorption
Antibiotics (broad spectrum)	Vitamin K, Biotin	Reduces endogenous vitamin production by colonic bacteria
Anticoagulants (warfarins)	Vitamin K	Antagonizes vitamin action
		High doses of vitamin K reduce the activity of the coumarins
	Vitamin E	High doses may potentiate anticoagulant action
Atropine	Iron	Reduces iron absorption
Azathioprine	Vitamin B6	Increases urinary B6 excretion
	Folate	Impairs folate metabolism
Barbiturates	Biotin, Vitamin B6, Vitamin B12, Riboflavin, Folate	Impairs vitamin metabolism and decreases serum levels
	Calcium	Reduces calcium absorption
	Vitamin D, Vitamin K	Increases vitamin breakdown and biliary excretion
	Vitamin C	Increases urinary vitamin C excretion
	Biotin	Decreases plasma biotin levels
	Potassium	Increases urinary potassium excretion
	Folate	High doses of folate may reverse the anticonvulsant effects
Beta-blockers	Niacin	High doses of niacin may enhance hypotensive action

Drug	Micronutrient	Interaction
Butyrophenone	Niacin, Manganese	Impairs vitamin metabolism
Calcitonin	Vitamin C	Increases vitamin requirement
	Magnesium	Reduces urinary magnesium excretion
	Calcium	Decreases calcium release from bone
Carbamazine	Biotin, Folate, Vitamin B12	Increases vitamin requirements
Carbenoxolone	Potassium	Increases urinary potassium excretion
Carbutamide	Potassium	Increases urinary potassium excretion
Cephalosporins (e. g. Moxalactam)	Vitamin K	Impairs vitamin metabolism
Chlorambucil	Vitamin B6	Increases urinary B6 excretion
Chloramphenicol	Vitamin B12	Reduces B12 absorption
	Folate	Increases folate requirements
	Vitamin K, Biotin	Reduces endogenous vitamin production by colonic bacteria
	Vitamin B6	Increases urinary B6 excretion
Chlorpromazine	Riboflavin	Increases urinary riboflavin excretion and impairs metabolism
Cholesterol-lowering drugs		
Cholestyramine	Vitamin A, Vitamin D, Vitamin E, Vitamin K, and Beta-carotene, Calcium, Magnesium, Folate, Vitamin B12, Iron	Reduces vitamin and mineral absorption

Drug	Micronutrient	Interaction
Cholesterol-lowering drugs		
	Calcium	Increases urinary calcium excretion
Colestipol	Vitamin A, Beta-carotene, Vitamin D, Vitamin E, Vitamin K, Calcium, Magnesium	Reduces vitamin and mineral absorption, lowers plasma levels of vitamins A and E
Clofibrate	Vitamin B12, Beta-carotene, Iron	Reduces vitamin and mineral absorption
HMG-CoA reductase inhibitors	Coenzyme Q10	Impairs CoQ10 metabolism
cis-Platinum	Potassium, Magnesium	Increases urinary mineral excretion
Colchicine	Vitamin A, Vitamin D, Vitamin E, Vitamin K, Vitamin B12, Beta-carotene	Reduces vitamin absorption
	Magnesium	Increases urinary magnesium excretion
Corticosteroids	Vitamin C	Increases vitamin C turnover and urinary excretion
	Vitamin B6	Increases B6 urinary excretion
	Folate	Impairs folate metabolism
	Vitamin D	Increases vitamin D requirement
	Calcium, Phosphorus	Reduces mineral absorption and increases urinary excretion
	Magnesium, Potassium, Zinc	Increases urinary mineral excretion
Cyclophosphamide	Vitamin B6	Increases urinary B6 excretion
Cycloserine	Folate, Vitamin B12	Impairs vitamin metabolism
	Vitamin B6	Impairs B6 metabolism and increases urinary excretion

Drug	Micronutrient	Interaction
Digitalis	Potassium, Magnesium	Increases urinary mineral excretion
Dimercaprol	Zinc, Copper	Increases urinary mineral excretion
DMSO (dimethyl sulfoxide)	Zinc, Copper	Increases urinary mineral excretion
Doxorubicin	Vitamin E	Increases vitamin E oxidation
Ethosuximide	Vitamin D	Impairs vitamin metabolism
Fiber (e. g. psyllium, bran)	Beta-carotene, Riboflavin, Zinc, Iron, Copper, Manganese	Reduces vitamin and mineral absorption
5-Fluorouracil	Thiamin	Reduces thiamin absorption
Glutethimide	Vitamin D	Increases vitamin requirement
Guanethidine	Niacin	Niacin enhances hypotensive action
Guanidine	Vitamin B12	Reduces B12 absorption
H_2-blockers	Vitamin B12, Iron	Reduces vitamin and mineral absorption
Hydralazine	Folate	Impairs folate metabolism
	Vitamin B6	Increases urinary B6 excretion
Indomethacin	Vitamin C	Decreases plasma and leukocyte vitamin levels
Insulin	Chromium	Chromium enhances hypoglycemic action
Isoniazid	Vitamin D	Impairs vitamin D metabolism
	Vitamin B6	Impairs vitamin B6 metabolism and increases urinary excretion
	Folate	Increases folate requirement
	Niacin	Reduces convesion of tryptophan to niacin
	Zinc	Increases urinary zinc excretion

Drug	Micronutrient	Interaction
Potassium chloride	Vitamin B12	Reduces vitamin B12 absorption
Kaolin	Riboflavin	Reduces riboflavin absorption
Ketoconazole	Magnesium	Reduces absorption of Ketoconazole
Oral contraceptives (estrogen-progesterone combinations)		
High-dose estrogen	Vitamin C	Increases vitamin C oxidation and decreases levels in plasma and leukocytes
	Vitamin B6, Riboflavin, Folate	Impairs vitamin metabolism
	Calcium	Increases calcium absorption
	Manganese, Zinc	Reduces blood mineral levels
	Carotenoids	Increases conversion to vitamin A
High and low-dose estrogen	Tryptophan	Increases conversion to niacin
	Vitamin A, Iron, Copper	Elevated vitamin and mineral levels in blood
Laxatives	Most vitamins and minerals	Reduces vitamin and mineral absorption due to accelerated transit time
Lithium	Magnesium, Potassium	Increases blood mineral levels
	Iodine	Impairs iodine metabolism
L-dopa	Vitamin B6	Decreases L-dopa activity
Loop diuretics (e. g. Lasix)	Potassium, Magnesium	Increases urinary mineral excretion
Mecamylamine	Magnesium	Reduces urinary excretion of mecamylamine
	Niacin	Niacin potentiates hypotensive effects

Drug	Micronutrient	Interaction
Mercaptopurine	Pantothenic acid	Impairs pantothenic acid metabolism
	Zinc	Increases zinc requirement
Metformin	Vitamin B12	Reduces vitamin absorption
	Folate	Decreases serum folate level
Methotrexate	Folate, Riboflavin Vitamin B12, Folate, Essential fatty acids	Impairs vitamin metabolism Reduces vitamin and fatty acid absorption
	Zinc	Increases zinc requirement
Mineral oil (laxative)	Vitamin A, Vitamin D, Vitamin E, Vitamin K, and Beta-carotene	Reduces vitamin absorption
Muscle relaxants	Thiamin	May enhance relaxant effect
Nitrofurantoin	Folate	Reduces folate absorption
Nitrous oxide	Vitamin B12	Increases B12 breakdown
Neomycin	Vitamin A, Vitamin D, Vitamin E, Vitamin K, Beta-carotene, Vitamin B12, Potassium, Calcium, Iron	Reduces vitamin and mineral absorption
	Vitamin K, Biotin	Reduces endogenous vitamin production by colonic bacteria
	Magnesium	Increases urinary magnesium excretion
Neuroleptics	Thiamin	Reduces thiamin absorption and increases excretion
Estrogen replacement therapy	Vitamin D	Increases synthesis of 1,25 $(OH)_2$ Vit D
	Calcium	Increases calcium absorption and decreases urinary excretion
	Vitamin B6	Impairs vitamin B6 metabolism

Drug	Micronutrient	Interaction
p-Aminosalicyl-saure	Vitamin B12, Folate, Iron	Reduces vitamin and mineral absorption
	Potassium	Increases urinary potassium excretion
Pargyline	Niacin	Niacin enhances hypotensive action
Penicillamine	Vitamin B6	Impairs B6 metabolism and increases urinary excretion
	Copper, Zinc	Increases urinary mineral excretion
Penicillin	Potassium	Increases urinary potassium excretion
Pentamidine	Folate	Impairs folate metabolism
Phenothiazine	Manganese	Increases excretion of manganese
	Riboflavin	Impairs riboflavin metabolism and increases urinary excretion
Phenylbutazone	Potassium	Increases urinary potassium excretion
	Folate	Impairs folate utilization
Phenytoin	Folate	Reduces absorption and impairs metabolism, high doses of folate antagonize anticonvulsive effects
	Vitamin B12	Decreases serum and brain levels
	Magnesium	Decreases serum magnesium levels
	Vitamin D, Vitamin K	Increases vitamin turnover
	Vitamin B6	High doses of B6 increase catabolism
	Calcium	Reduces calcium absorption
	Zinc	Increases zinc requirement
	Copper	Increases serum copper level

Drug	Micronutrient	Interaction
Potassium-sparing diuretics (Spironolactone, Triamterene)	Folate	Impairs metabolism
	Potassium, Magnesium	Reduces urinary mineral excretion
Primidone	Folate	Impairs metabolism and reduces absorption, high doses of folate antagonize effects
	Vitamin B6, Vitamin B12	Decreases serum vitamin levels
	Vitamin D, Vitamin K	Increases vitamin breakdown and excretion
	Calcium	Reduces calcium absorption
Probenecid	Riboflavin	Reduces riboflavin absorption
	Calcium, Magnesium, Potassium	Increases urinary mineral excretion
Pyrimethamine	Folate, Vitamin B12	Impairs vitamin metabolism, folate antagonizes activity
Quinidine	Vitamin K	Impairs vitamin K status
Quinine	Folate	Impairs folate status
Rifampicin	Vitamin D	Increases vitamin D turnover
	Calcium	Reduces calcium absorption due to decreased activity of vitamin D
Salicylates	Vitamin A, Vitamin B6	Reduces vitamin clearance
	Vitamin C	Reduces vitamin C absorption, decreases uptake into leukocytes and levels in plasma and platelets; increases urinary excretion
	Vitamin K	Impairs vitamin metabolism

Drug	Micronutrient	Interaction
Salicylates	Iron	Increases iron losses from the digestive tract
	Folate	Decreases serum folate levels
Salazosulfapyridine	Folate	Reduces folate absorption and impairs metabolism
Sodium nitroprusside	Vitamin B12	Increases urinary vitamin B12 excretion
Sulfonamide	Folate	Impairs folate metabolism
Sulfonylureas	Niacin	High doses of niacin may reduce the effectiveness of certain oral hypoglycemic drugs
Tetracycline	Vitamin C	Impairs vitamin C metabolism and increases urinary excretion
	Magnesium, Zinc, Calcium, Iron	Reduces both mineral and tetracycline absorption
	Zinc	Increases urinary excretion
	Vitamin K, Biotin	Reduces endogenous vitamin production by colonic bacteria
	Riboflavin, Vitamin C	Increases urinary vitamin excretion
Thiazides	Vitamin B-complex, Vitamin C, Potassium, Magnesium, Zinc	Increases urinary vitamin and mineral excretion
	Calcium	Decreases urinary calcium excretion
Theophylline	Vitamin B6	Impairs vitamin metabolism
Thyroxine	Riboflavin	Reduces riboflavin absorption
	Vitamin E	Impairs vitamin metabolism
Trimethoprim	Folate	Impairs folate metabolism and reduces absorption
Valproic acid	Copper, Zinc, Selenium	Reduces serum mineral levels

References

Handbook on Drug and Nutrient Interactions. Chicago: American Dietetic Association; 1994.
Knapp H. Nutrient–drug interactions. In: Ziegler EE, Filer LJ, eds. Present Knowledge in Nutrition. Washington DC: ILSI Press; 1996.
Roe DA. Diet, nutrition, and drug reactions. In: Shils ME, Olson JA, Shike M, eds. Modern Nutrition in Health and Disease. Philadelphia: Lea & Febiger; 1994.
Thomas JA. Drug–nutrient interactions. Nutr Rev. 1995;53:271.

Nutrient–Nutrient Interactions

Nutrient		Interaction
Calcium (Ca)	Magnesium	High doses reduce Ca absorption, deficiency produces hypocalcemia
	Phosphorus	High intakes (> 2 g/day) increase urinary excretion of Ca
	Protein	High intakes increase urinary excretion of Ca
	Sodium	Increases urinary Ca excretion
	Vitamin D	Promotes Ca absorption and Ca release from the skeleton; decreases urinary excretion of Ca
	Zinc	High intakes (> 140 mg/day) reduce Ca absorption
Carnitine	Vitamin C	Deficiency increases carnitine requirements
Chromium (Cr)	Calcium	High doses of Ca carbonate reduce Cr absorption
	Iron	Iron deficiency enhances Cr absorption. Saturating blood transferrin with iron reduces blood Cr transport and retention
Copper (Cu)	Cadmium	Impairs Cu absorption and utilization
	Iron	Large doses reduce Cu absorption
	Molybdenum	Increases Cu urinary excretion
	Vitamin B6	Deficiency decreases Cu absorption
	Vitamin C	High levels decrease Cu absorption and reduce levels of ceruloplasmin, may stimulate Cu utilization
	Zinc	High doses (> 80 mg/day) reduce Cu absorption
Fluoride (F)	Calcium	Reduces F absorption

Nutrient		Interaction
Folic acid	Vitamin B12	Deficiency impairs folate utilization and metabolism
	Niacin	Deficiency reduces activation of folate
	Vitamin C	Maintains body stores of folate and reduces urinary folate excretion
Iron (Fe)	Calcium	Reduces absorption of both heme and non-heme Fe
	Copper	High doses reduce Fe absorption, deficiency impairs utilization of body Fe
	Manganese	Reduces Fe absorption
	Riboflavin	Deficiency may reduce Fe absorption, impair Fe metabolism, and increase risk of anemia
	Vitamin A	Deficiency impairs mobilization and utilization of body Fe, and plasma Fe levels fall
	Vitamin B6	Deficiency impairs Fe metabolism
	Vitamin E	May reduce hematologic response to Fe in treatment of Fe-deficiency anemia
	Vitamin C	Sharply increases absorption of Fe and overcomes inhibition of Fe absorption by phenols and phytates, enhances Fe utilization by tissues
	Zinc	Reduces Fe absorption
Magnesium (Mg)	Calcium	High doses reduce Mg absorption hypercalcema increases urinary Mg excretion, while hypocalcemia reduces urinary Mg excretion
	Iron	Reduces Mg absorption
	Manganese	Reduces Mg absorption
	Phosphorus	Reduces Mg absorption. Deficiency increases urinary Mg excretion
	Potassium	Increases urinary Mg excretion
	Sodium	Increases urinary Mg excretion
	Vitamin B6	Increases intracellular Mg levels and utilization

Nutrient		Interaction
	Vitamin E	Deficiency decreases tissue levels of Mg
	Vitamin D	Enhances bioavailability of Mg
Manganese (Mn)	Calcium	Reduces Mn absorption
	Copper	Reduces Mn absorption
	Phosphate	Reduces Mn absorption
	Iron	Reduces Mn absorption and impairs utilization
	Vitamin C	May increase Mn bioavailability
Molybdenum (Mo)	Copper	High doses interfere with Mo metabolism
Niacin	Tryptophan	Precursor in niacin synthesis
	Riboflavin	Essential cofactor in synthesis of niacin from trytophan; deficiency will impair synthesis of niacin
	Vitamin B6	Essential cofactor in synthesis of niacin from trytophan; deficiency will impair synthesis of niacin
Omega-6 fatty acids (evening primrose oil, GLA)	Omega-3 fatty acids	Increasing intake will reduce utilization of omega-6 fatty acids
	Vitamin E	Reduces peroxidation of essential fatty acids
Omega-3 fatty acids (fish oils, EPA, DHA)	Omega-6 fatty acids	Increasing intake will reduce utilization of omega-3 fatty acids
	Vitamin E	Reduces peroxidation of essential fatty acids in tissues
Potassium (K)	Magnesium	Deficiency increases urinary K excretion
Riboflavin	Niacin	Important in the activation of riboflavin
Selenium (Se)	Vitamin C	Deficiency impairs Se utilization, high doses reduce absorption of inorganic forms of Se (such as sodium selenite)

Nutrient		Interaction
	Vitamin E	Deficiency increases Se requirement
Thiamine	Magnesium	Deficiency impairs activation of thiamin to thiamin pyrophosphate
	Vitamin C	Protects thiamin from inactivation in the GI tract by polyphenols
	Folic acid	Deficiency reduces absorption of thiamin
Tryptophan	Protein	When consumed with tryptophan supplements reduces brain tryptophan levels, because dietary amino acids compete with tryptophan for transport into the brain
	Carbohydrate	When consumed with tryptophan supplements increases brain tryptophan levels, because insulin secretion in response to carbohydrate promotes transport of competing amino acids out of bloodstream, increasing tryptophan uptake into the brain
	Vitamin B6	High doses increase brain tryptophan levels
Vitamin A	Vitamin C	May reduce toxicity from vitamin A
	Vitamin E	Enhances the absorption, storage, and utilization of vitamin A; reduces the toxic effects of high doses of vitamin A
	Zinc	Deficiency impairs vitamin A metabolism and utilization
Vitamin B6	Niacin	Important in the activation of vitamin B6
	Riboflavin	Important in the conversion of vitamin B6 to active forms
	Zinc	Important in the conversion of vitamin B6 to active forms
	Vitamin C	Deficiency may increase vitamin B6 urinary excretion
Vitamin B12	Potassium (chloride)	Extended release KCl tablets reduce vitamin B12 absorption
	Folic acid	Large doses may mask hematologic signs of vitamin B12 deficiency

Nutrient		Interaction
Vitamin C	Iron	Large doses reduce blood vitamin C levels through oxidation
	Vitamin A	Chronic high doses may reduce tissue levels of vitamin C and increase urinary exretion
	Vitamin B6	Deficiency may increase risk of vitamin C deficiency
Vitamin D	Vitamin E	Deficiency impairs vitamin D metabolism
	Magnesium	Deficiency impairs vitamin D activity
	Calcium	Hypocalcemia stimulates vitamin D conversion to active forms; hypercalcemia inhibits vitamin D activation
	Phosphorus	Hypophosphatemia stimulates vitamin D conversion to active forms; hyperphosphatemia inhibits vitamin D activation
Vitamin E	Iron	Large doses increase requirement for vitamin E
	Copper	Large doses increase requirement for vitamin E
	Zinc	Deficiency reduces vitamin E blood levels
	Selenium	Poor status increases requirement for vitamin E
	Vitamin C	Reduces oxidized tocopherol back to active tocopherol, thereby conserving vitamin E stores
	Essential fatty acids	Increases requirement for vitamin E
Vitamin K	Calcium	High doses of Ca, or a dietary Ca: phosphorus ratio > 2:1 may impair vitamin K status
	Vitamin E	Large doses (> 1200 mg/day) may reduce absorption and activity of vitamin K
	Vitamin A	High doses reduce absorption of vitamin K, and hypothrombinemia may occur

Nutrient		Interaction
Zinc (Zn)	Calcium	High doses reduce Zn absorption
	Copper	Reduces Zn absorption
	Folic acid	Reduces Zn absorption
	Iron	When the iron/Zn ratio in the diet is > 2:1, absorption of Zn is impaired
	Cysteine	Enhances Zn absorption
	Histidine	Enhances Zn absorption
	Vitamin A	Enhances Zn absorption
	Vitamin B6	Enhances Zn absorption; vitamin B6 deficiency reduces plasma Zn levels
	Vitamin E	Deficiency reduces plasma Zn levels and may exacerbate Zn deficiency

Index

D

E

I

K

L

R

S

T

U

V